living well with depression

Also Available for Professionals

Behavioral Activation for Depression:
A Clinician's Guide, Second Edition

Christopher R. Martell, Sona Dimidjian, and Ruth Herman-Dunn

Behavioral Activation with Adolescents: A Clinician's Guide

Elizabeth McCauley, Kelly A. Schloredt, Gretchen R. Gudmundsen, Christopher R. Martell, and Sona Dimidjian

Cognitive-Behavioral Therapies with Lesbian, Gay, and Bisexual Clients

Christopher R. Martell, Steven A. Safren, and Stacey E. Prince

Praise for **Living Well with Depression**

"I appreciate Dr. Martell's easy-to-understand suggestions and advice; handy checklists; and calm, reassuring tone. This is a book you can turn to whenever you hit a depression roadblock and need help finding your way to a better place."

—Bruce C., Amherst, Massachusetts

"If depression is affecting your daily life, this book is for you. Dr. Martell has spent decades studying depression and helping people recover. This book offers nitty-gritty tools and guidance to cope with issues that even the best treatments can't always address."

—Jacqueline B. Persons, PhD, Director, Oakland Cognitive Behavior Therapy Center

"As someone with intermittent depression (and a health care professional), I have finally found a book that addresses the ups and downs of living with depression and its impact on everyday functioning. I love Dr. Martell's explanation of 'acting from the outside in' and his simple recommendations—for example, if you can't get out of bed, try just putting your feet on the floor."

—Georgia M., Bennington, Vermont

"This is a book I want for my clients, but also for my friends. The book is filled with practical tips; can be taken in small, manageable pieces; and is a lovely complement to therapy."

—Debra Kaysen, PhD, ABPP, Department of Psychiatry and Behavioral Sciences, Stanford University

"Dr. Martell helps you develop routines that stabilize your mood, and the focus on working on one thing at time prevents you from feeling overwhelmed. I especially appreciate the advice about living in the present and experiencing the sights, sounds, and other senses of the world around us."

—Ann K., Hinesburg, Vermont

"Dr. Martell is a world-renowned depression expert who presents clear, compassionate, highly practical strategies to help you navigate real-world challenges and live well. Drawing on effective evidence-based treatments, this book is exceptionally useful and empowering."

—Steven A. Safren, PhD, ABPP, Department of Psychology, University of Miami

THE GUILFORD LIVING WELL SERIES

The Guilford Living Well Series is designed to help individuals with common psychological conditions solve everyday problems and optimize their quality of life. Readers get specific, empathic advice for stress-proofing daily routines; navigating work, family, and relationship issues; managing symptoms effectively; and finding answers to treatment questions. Written by leading experts on each disorder, books in the series are concise, practical, and empowering.

Living Well with Bipolar Disorder
David J. Miklowitz

Living Well with OCD
Jonathan S. Abramowitz

Living Well with Psychosis
Aaron P. Brinen

Living Well with Adult ADHD
Laura E. Knouse and Russell A. Barkley

Living Well with Social Anxiety
Deborah Dobson

Living Well with Depression
Christopher R. Martell

FORTHCOMING

Living Well When Food Is an Issue
Rhonda M. Merwin

living well *with* depression

PRACTICAL STRATEGIES FOR IMPROVING YOUR DAILY LIFE

CHRISTOPHER R. MARTELL, PhD

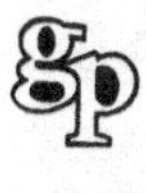

THE GUILFORD PRESS
NEW YORK   LONDON

A Division of Guilford Publications, Inc.
www.guilford.com

Printed in the United States of America

For product and safety concerns within the EU, please contact *GPSR@taylorandfrancis.com,* Taylor & Francis Verlag GmbH, Kaufingerstraße 24, 80331 München, Germany.

Last digit is print number: 9 8 7 6 5 4 3 2 1

Library of Congress Cataloging-in-Publication Data

Names: Martell, Christopher R. author
Title: Living well with depression : practical strategies for improving your daily life / Christopher R. Martell, PhD.
Description: New York : The Guilford Press, [2026] | Series: The Guilford living well series | Includes bibliographical references and index.
Identifiers: LCCN 2026020367 | ISBN 9781462553860 paperback | ISBN 9781462563982 hardcover
Subjects: LCSH: Depression, Mental | Self-actualization (Psychology) | LCGFT: Self-help publications
Classification: LCC RC537 .M37375 2026
LC record available at *https://lccn.loc.gov/2026020367*

contents

Purchasers of this book can download and print additional copies of the forms in this book at *www.guilford.com/martell3-materials* for personal use or use with clients (see copyright page for details).

living well with depression

introduction

A DAY IN THE LIFE OF DEPRESSION

Depression is tough to live with. That's because, even when treatment has helped, you may feel as if you haven't returned to your usual self and you're not living the full life you once enjoyed. William Styron, the author of *Sophie's Choice,* called depression "darkness visible" in his memoir for good reason.[1] For many people, depression dampens joy and makes daily activities a little more difficult, even when symptoms have improved.

There are plenty of books on how to assess and diagnose depression, and how to treat it or prevent it. You have probably read some of them. And yet, here you are—likely because there are few resources designed to support people like you who may find depression is always operational in some form. You may be in treatment but still struggle to make it through the day. You might feel as if you don't have any agency in your own life, that everything feels bleak and joyless, and that can be a discouraging feeling.

Or perhaps you're experiencing your first episode right now. If so, you likely feel as if you've become a different person. You may no longer trust that the aspects of your life that have brought you joy so far will ever do so again.

If depression is recurrent for you, you may worry about what you'll experience if the darkness is starting to overtake you again. Perhaps you're starting to realize that your "normal" state may be to always be at least a little depressed. We used to call this "dysthymia;" now we call it *persistent depression*. If this is your diagnosis, you may not fathom what it would mean for you to live well, because your mood is never expansive, and joy is often elusive.

To complicate things further, daily life with depression looks different for different people. Mathematically, there are 126 different ways to meet depression criteria in the DSM-5,[2] although making diagnoses is not a matter of mathematics. The point here is that "depression" isn't just one thing for everyone. Depression is a cluster of "symptoms" or experiences that are common.

You may experience intense negative emotions like sadness and feelings of hopelessness. You may not really feel anything at all. You may be living in a continual state of brain fog and have difficulty concentrating, or you may have a busy brain that won't shut off with thoughts about past mistakes, hurts, or losses.

You're very likely avoiding engaging in any activities that could possibly give you pleasure. And if you were to do something you used to enjoy, you would probably feel as though it were meaningless. There are nearly infinite ways that people are affected by depression.

And, fortunately, there are as many ways that you can prevent depression from having such a strong hold on your life. This book shares multiple ways to help you lead a more fulfilling life despite having symptoms of depression.

Who This Book Is For

This book is for you if you're living with depression in any of the ways described so far. As difficult as it may seem at times, I encourage you to hold on to hope that your depression will lift, that help you are seeking will work, that you can live well, and that depression need not conquer you. I've crafted this book to give you that hope. As I've seen in my work treating people living with depression or training other therapists around the world to do so, you *can* live well with depression, even if the negative feelings don't go away, or if you don't experience the same pleasures as you once did.

In the following pages, you'll find practical strategies that can make daily life easier and ideally more pleasurable. Some of them will be new to you, even if you have received professional treatment and read popular self-help books. Others will be familiar, but in this book I'll show you how to modify techniques or use them in new ways so they support you right where you are. You can begin to live well right now, whether that darkness lifts or you just need to do something other than white-knuckle it through the gloom.

The suggestions are practical, and therefore look simple. However, applying even the simplest strategies when you're depressed can be extremely difficult. To quote Styron again, "To most of those who have experienced it, the horror of depression is so overwhelming as to be quite beyond expression."[3] Even taking the smallest step with any of the suggestions in this book can begin a journey to living well—either out of depression, or *with* it.

Therapies That Inform This Book

Living Well with Depression is not intended to be a therapy self-help book. There are plenty of those in publication and many are good. Nor is it meant as a replacement for therapy. Instead, this book is designed to be a menu of strategies you can choose for a variety of challenging daily situations. The many strategies on offer are used in a range of therapies that have proven *efficacy,* or effectiveness, in many rigorous scientific studies.

Some techniques will work, others may not. As a clinical psychologist who has worked with clients for more than 30 years, I've learned that even the best therapies with the most elegant strategies land differently with different people. Some aspects of a treatment really resonate with clients, or make sense to them at a very particular time in their lives. Others don't work for some people—and if that has been the case for you, it is because not every strategy, nor every therapist for that matter, is a good fit for every person. In this book, I'm offering the best strategies from these well researched therapies. It's up to you to try them and discover which will help you get through the day.

Should you find that seeking professional help would suit you, the following therapies provide the bases for the suggestions and ideas presented in this book. There are likely therapists in your geographic region or online who work from one or a combination of these approaches. These are not the only approaches to psychotherapy. They are listed here because it is from these therapies that the suggestions in this book have derived. This book in no way claims to be a comprehensive presentation of any of the therapies shared.

Cognitive-Behavioral Therapy

The name says it all, with "cognitive" referring to the way you think and "behavioral" referring to the way you act. *Cognitive-behavioral therapy* (CBT) is based on the premise that our emotions, thoughts, behaviors, and biology are all connected, and changes in any of these areas affect the others. In this way, it takes a holistic view of people. The strategies derived from this perspective help you to identify your reactions (thoughts, behaviors, physical sensations, and feelings) to life events and then evaluate helpful and unhelpful responses. The goals of CBT are to change how you feel by changing how you think and act.[4]

Behavioral Activation

Behavioral activation (BA)[5] is a particular model of the broader CBT approaches. It is a behavioral treatment for depression and one that I have written about extensively. The premise of BA is that changing how you act can change how you feel; likewise, when your feelings *don't* change, you can still act in ways that make your life better. The process is to identify your goals; break down steps to your goals; identify what's blocking you from reaching your goals; and find ways to overcome those barriers. In BA, we look at thoughts in the same way as we look at observable behaviors, but we recognize that they are private to the person. We consider the *process* of your thinking, and less about the *content* of your thoughts.

Acceptance and Commitment Therapy

Acceptance and commitment therapy (ACT)[6] is a newer behavioral therapy. In the ACT approach there is a focus on *values-guided* or *values-consistent* action, which means maneuvering life's challenges by what matters most to you. Dr. Steve Hayes, one of the developers of ACT, has said ACT is about how to "get out of your mind and into your life," which happens to be the title of one of his books (see the online companion Resources page at *www.guilford.com/martell3-materials*).

Interpersonal Therapies

Interpersonal therapies (IPT)[7] focus on how interpersonal histories may still be impacting you today. It involves looking at how your current interpersonal interactions and networks can impact your mood, or your ability to live well. The need to understand how your relationships affect you and how to build a good network (even if that network is one or two people) is important.

How This Book Can Help

If actual treatment hasn't been fully successful, why would a book help? My aim is to offer suggestions for what you can do in the moment to give you a little boost in your mood or keep you going—every day, in all kinds of typical situations, from getting out of bed to dealing with a difficult family member to taking steps to move forward in a career. The strategies derive from three overarching principles:

1. *Allow your emotions*
2. *Be proactive*
3. *Think flexibly*

Habit, routine, and normal patterns help us maintain our emotional balance when the world challenges us and our lives are thrown off kilter. Also, that is where change begins, in developing new habits.

The goal is to allow your emotions to exist (while not necessarily basing your immediate actions on them), to get better at making behavioral changes a permanent part of your life. This is true also of the goal to think more flexibly. These goals may sound simple, and yet they're terribly hard to practice without a little guidance. I will provide that in these pages.

Everything in this book is written to be a hand that helps lift you up, little by little. The ideas are meant to change your relationship to your emotions, change your behavior, and change the way you think about the world, yourself, and the future—also known as changing your relationship to your thoughts.

The depressed mind can be filled with scary thoughts about never feeling good again, or about how you once enjoyed life but now there is nothing that you care about or enjoy. Those powerful thoughts are a trap. The more you think about how depressed you feel, the more depressed you will be, and the more you will act from the depressed mood.

It sounds strange to consider living well with depression when you've experienced the bleakness of it. But science tells us that desperately wanting moods to go away only increases the pain, like trying to pull your leg out of a bear trap; without a key to open it, you will just hurt more. The hope is that you will find a key, or several keys, in these pages to getting out of the depression trap.

How to Navigate This Book

You might want to read this book from beginning to end, but it doesn't need to be used this way. Part One introduces the three principles for living well with depression. You might wish to read this in its entirety for a foundation. Part Two extends the principles to situations in everyday life. It begins with a chapter offering suggestions for considering what is most important to you—your values, relationships, and overall outlook on life. The remaining chapters in Part Two address common situations that people often find challenging, particularly when they are living with depression. These chapters can serve as independent units—dishes on a menu, if you will—that you can turn to when you are in similar situations. Along the way I'll introduce some characters who are entirely fictional or have some composite concerns of people I've known or treated (with identifying features disguised or fictional).

Healing Begins with Hope

I always recommend that the best place to start—and this is really important—is with hope. You've picked up this book, so you likely have hope that there is something in these pages that might be of use to you. You're right! You don't need motivation, or high energy, or excitement to live well and to benefit from some of the strategies in this book. You do need *hope,* but it can be only a faint glimmer. All you need is a small, vulnerable, and tenuous desire to find something that will be helpful, and that you will find it within these pages.

PART ONE

three principles to live well with depression

1

emotions

ALLOW YOUR FEELINGS

Emotions are as much a part of you as is any physical feeling. Sometimes you will wake up with a sore neck or a tummy ache, and sometimes you will feel angry or worried. You can't always feel happy, and you can't completely run away from emotional pain. Fighting against your feelings usually only makes you feel worse. So, the first step in living well with depression is to allow the feelings and be patient with the process, even if it feels like you're just going through the motions.

What Is an Emotion?

Emotions are the fluctuating feelings that color our lives, usually connected to something that has happened during the day; some thoughts or memories we've been brooding on; some unknown physical cause; or even from having had a night of bad dreams that we don't recall. We get scared if we hear a loud noise, mad when someone makes a rude gesture on the freeway, and so forth.

A *mood* is a longer-lasting experience or a general state of being. We experience moods as more systemic; they can last a whole day or feel almost eternal. The American Psychological Association metaphorically describes moods as climate and emotions as the temperature.

For instance, a winter climate is generally cold, rainy, or snowy (the mood) while the temperature (the emotion) can fluctuate, from 30 degrees one day to 55 the next. With depression, it's not uncommon for people to think of it as both a mood (a long-term condition) *and* a feeling (temporary).

To live well with depression is to live well with the mood aspect, allowing the full spectrum of emotions to be present, even when your predominant mood may be depressed. You will see in this book that what you *do* can have an impact on both your feelings and your mood. Different activities can make you feel more or less depressed. An important aspect of living well with depression is becoming aware of what you want to *keep* or even *increase* in your life, as well as what you want to do *less* of.

Why Do We Have Emotions?

Let's talk about "normal" emotions. From a holistic perspective, there are no "bad" emotions, although we humans can experience certain ones as hard. Every emotion has a function, and there are reasons that human beings evolved to have them. Here are some possible reasons that we have certain basic emotions:

- ***Fear.*** It keeps us out of harm's way. If you see a snake slither across your path, you likely have an automatic, immediate response to jump back away from it. When it's just a harmless garden snake, there is nothing you need protection from, but in some places in the world, and certainly when humans lived in less-protected environments than most do now, that fear response could be lifesaving. Some fears are almost innate, like the reflexive jumping away from something slithering in the grass, and some are developed over time through our own experiences or through modeling of others, particularly of our caretakers when we are children.
- ***Anxiety.*** If you have ever felt anxious or nervous before taking a test, or going on a job interview, or before introducing yourself to

someone new, you might wonder why you can't just be calm. However, all people feel anxiety in some situations. It serves us well. We need some level of anxiety to keep us aroused and working to do our best. It also protects us. If you were a parent of a young child and you had no anxiety, you would let your child play with broken glass or walk away with a stranger who took their hand in the park. Your apprehension in such circumstances serves you, and in this example, your child, well.

- ***Sadness.*** We feel sad when we have lost something or somebody important to us. Sadness lets your community know you are in need. It also can be a cue for you to self-soothe and have empathy for yourself. People actually seek sadness to some extent, such as a drive to watch tear-jerker movies—people get pulled into the empathy for the characters and the pathos.

- ***Depression.*** Evolutionary psychologists suggest that the experiences that we associate with symptoms of depression—like low energy, decreased motivation, and so forth—may have served humans in smaller communities by keeping the social order. It reduces our threat potential to others. If one of our human ancestors did not get to be leader of the community, they may have felt what we now would call disappointment. They may have felt fatigued, unmotivated, sad, or had the urge to shut down. How could that have been good? Well, it reduced the urge to force their way into leadership through brute strength and threat. Disappointment and sadness are very important for social animals.

Uma's Story

Uma just wanted to cry. But she thought that if she let herself go, the crying would last forever and she would not recover from the despair. It terrified her to always feel on the edge of crying. Uma knew she would not die from crying, but she worried that the tears would be relentless, showing up during conversations with others, keeping her from sleeping, pulling her deeper into a virtual crevasse of pain.

Eventually, she was able to lean into allowing herself to cry. She began by watching a sad movie that she had seen years before. She cried from the middle of the film to the end and then some, but the tears eventually stopped. Uma recognized that there was a release without being forever stuck, and that it actually felt helpful to cry and let out those pent-up feelings.

The ARC of Our Emotions

Psychologist David Barlow and his colleagues came up with an easy acronym to understand the features of an emotion: ARC.[1]

- **A:** *Antecedent,* or the situation or event that occurs
- **R:** *Response,* or the emotion we have as a reaction to the event
- **C:** *Consequence,* or what happens when we have a certain emotional response

Our emotional response (R) includes what our bodies feel. For example, you may get a feeling like a pit in your stomach when you feel anxious or scared, or you may feel tension, or maybe experience both.

The emotional response also consists of our thoughts and our behaviors. Cognitive-behavioral therapists frequently quote Shakespeare's *Hamlet* in saying, "There is nothing either good or bad, but thinking makes it so." In other words, we make interpretations of events and judgments. These interpretations can be accurate and helpful, accurate yet unhelpful, or inaccurate and unhelpful. In some instances an interpretation could be inaccurate yet helpful, for example interpreting someone's sneer as withholding a sneeze might prevent a feeling of anger, although they may have intended to indicate some displeasure. We don't need to change inaccurate interpretations that are helpful because they will usually be inconsequential. The thought, or "cognitive" aspect, of our emotional responses can be evaluated and changed; they're often what therapists help with. We'll talk more about our thoughts in relation to our emotions in Chapter 3.

Behaviors stem from the impulse to act as an immediate response to the event. Again, we've evolved this way. When walking in tall grass and something rushes past us, we instinctively jump back. Whether it turns out to be a snake, the wind, or a little field mouse, we jump. Even people who aren't afraid of snakes or mice or other slithery things will jump. It's the natural, automatic urge. These are evolved impulses, as well as a product of social convention, and our personal histories.

Some behaviors are helpful, like the urge to wade in cool water on a blistering hot day, and some are unhelpful, like the urge to avoid a shortcut when you're running late because you remember that once someone had an accident there. We'll talk more about our behaviors in response to our emotions in Chapter 2.

Managing how we respond to life events is a key to living well with depression. So much of the emotional response is either blunted, painful, or unhelpful when you're controlled by depressed mood. The task ahead is to recognize and welcome your emotions—or at least tolerate them. Minimizing unhelpful beliefs and behavior patterns while finding helpful ways to think and act are ongoing steps to living well.

What If We Don't Like Our Emotions?

You can't completely run away from emotional pain. If you have persistent depression, you know that you can numb the pain with sleep, distractions, or mind-altering substances, but they ultimately don't help, or they make things worse. Medications can help, but they aren't meant to remove all feelings and emotions.

Sometimes what you experience is an absence of emotions. When you are dealing with persistent depression, you may not feel excited or happy about many things. Fighting this sensation will only make you feel worse. So, the first step in living well with depression is to allow the feelings, even though it may seem as if you're going to be overwhelmed by them, and be patient with the process.

Research shows that, for most people, depression will lift after six months to a year; even when it is chronic, it's not always deep. You don't need to just tough it out. (Some research suggests that "watchful waiting" may be as helpful as receiving a prescription for antidepressant medication from a primary care provider, but there is conflicting data.[2]) The pain will not last interminably, although it may seem to you as if it will.

Likewise, as Dr. Gregory Scott Brown stated in a *Washington Post* article, "happiness can be fleeting."[3] You may often painfully notice that happiness is short-lived or hard to find, and regret about that can deepen a depressed mood. You may fear that hurtful emotions will never end. But in all seriousness, you won't cry forever and you won't be sad forever. Even if you wept incessantly for a long period of time, you would most likely fall into an exhausted sleep rather than drown in your tears. In other words, don't be afraid of feelings; whatever they are, they will ebb and flow.

It Doesn't Make You Weak to Feel Emotional

Culturally, you may express emotions in a certain way. You've also been culturally conditioned to feel emotions in a way that likely feels natural. We are also socialized to express feelings according to our sex or gender, in keeping with religious expectations, and so forth.

However, expressing emotions and feeling emotions may be different things. If you were to attend a funeral, for example, in a culture where men are expected not to cry but it is perfectly acceptable for women to be tearful, what might you observe? Even in this context, you're likely to see that some of the men are shedding tears, perhaps quietly; a few may be choking on them a little or frequently blowing their noses. Some women will wipe their eyes throughout, and others will sit stoically without shedding a tear. All of this is simply human variation. It would be inaccurate to think that the men who are crying are weaker than the men who are not, or that the women who aren't crying are heartless. Having emotions, feeling them, and expressing them in the way that is natural for you just *is,* and there is no need to judge strength or weakness.

It Doesn't Make You Strong to Hide Emotions

How you express emotions is not as important as *what* you express. Being the "strong, silent, type" is a myth. Strong people may not always outwardly express emotions, but they don't run from the discomfort of emotion. Likewise, being cast as "a robot" is not a fair depiction of anyone who doesn't show emotion naturally, even though they may feel them deeply.

Again, culture plays a role here, and so does your own history. Within the confines of what is consistent with cultural standards that you agree with, you don't need to stuff emotions and hide them away. You may express them by simply asserting that you feel a certain way, like calmly telling someone they have offended you, or you may tearfully say that you have been hurt by another's actions.

The point here is that intentionally hiding emotions (or the reverse, putting on an inauthentic show for the sake of others; see next paragraph) doesn't make you strong or noble, it just means you aren't allowing yourself to be yourself. Allow emotions to be part of your life.

It Doesn't Make You Interesting to Show Your Emotions to Everyone

There is the expression that some people "wear their emotions on their sleeves." While it's not helpful to run away and try not to feel emotion, it also is not helpful to act on every *action urge* connected with the emotional response. (We will discuss action urges more in Chapter 2.) Showing your emotion to everyone around you can turn others away. Reacting too strongly or dramatically can be as socially unhelpful as staying emotionally blunted. The over-feeling of emotions can also cause you more suffering, just like the under-feeling of emotions can.

Changing Your Relationship to Your Emotions

Having painful emotions is not the problem; it's how you manage them that can get you into trouble. Yet how do you manage emotions when they feel so out of your control; when you feel as if you are managed by them; when you may be vulnerable to extremely low moods or volatile emotions? It's not your fault—you cannot take blame for not being able to completely control moods and emotions or (in some cases) the lack of emotion.

However, you can look at emotions as a part of yourself that you can have a relationship with. You can start by stepping back and observing what you feel, what you believe about what you feel, and what your emotions pull you to do. Consider some common thoughts about emotions that people have:

"I feel as if this depression will last forever."

Some people feel that their feelings, particularly during depressed moods, have always been there and will always be there. That feeling can be strong, and there are several reasons for that. When emotions are strong, our thought processes are affected. When we are depressed, our memories can be clouded by the depression. We remember having struggled with depressed moods for all of our lives, and then we feel as though we've been *depressed* for our entire lives. It's hard to see any future but a depressed future, because we believe that the strong moods and emotions of today will always be the same.

For most people, depressed moods or a "major depressive episode" will last some weeks. Seeking therapy can be helpful to manage this period of time, particularly when the mood lasts longer. You may be someone who experiences chronic depression, and in this case, the depression can last even longer. Even so, you don't have to suffer forever.

RATE YOUR BLUES

Not every unhappy mood is created equal. Sometimes you might feel a little bit down, other days or hours of the day you might feel simply dreadful. So, it's good to understand the various intensities of your moods. Rating your moods and keeping track of them can give you credible data about times when you feel worse, along with when you feel better. When you see that your moods change, you can use this data to remind yourself that particularly bad patches don't last forever, that you're not completely stuck. Even brief periods of feeling differently—enjoying a phone conversation, smiling at seeing a cute animal play in your yard—tell you that you can live well as these moments increase over time.

1 2 3 4 5 6 7 8 9 10

Rate your moods throughout the day, keeping track of them in a journal or notes app on your phone. Think of 10 as the most depressed you've felt and 1 as least depressed.

"I don't feel anything."

We may also feel flat, neither sad nor happy, as if we don't care. Mental health professionals call this *anhedonia.* Anhedonia likely has some degree of neurobiological basis within the brain's reward system. It doesn't mean that we are inherently unfeeling or uncaring. It's more about life seeming dull and colorless. With it can come a downward cycle of not feeling like doing anything, then doing nothing, and then feeling even less like doing anything. It's hard to engage in life when you don't experience emotions. But there are some tricks to get out of the cycle.

ACT FROM THE OUTSIDE IN

Most people have heard the expression "fake it 'til you make it." I prefer to use the expression *acting from the outside in.* This means relying on external aids rather than on your mood. Breaking the habit of acting according to your mood is the point here.

To me, it's all about *making it,* not faking it. Don't pretend to feel one way or another; simply *act according to a plan,* or in a way consistent with your values. *Acting from the outside in* means following a plan that you develop, committing to what you will do. Over time, it can actually change how you feel.

The dilemma of feeling unmotivated to do the very things that are in line with our goals, or that fit with our values and what's important, keeps many people stuck. Equally problematic is when we follow "positive" feelings, and they pull us away from what we value. One of the most common examples of that may be when people who highly value family and stability follow their emotions and cheat on a partner. Fortunately, there are strategies that can help people out of this dilemma by acting from the outside in.

Any activity can lift your mood, though it isn't likely to happen suddenly. If that were possible, we could walk off all of our concerns. Committing to repetition will give you successful experiences and impact your mood over time. Here's what you can do:

1. Write down at least two activities that are aligned with your goals rather than your mood. They need to be something that you can engage in every day and that you can do regardless of how you feel, what the weather is like, or how busy your day is.
2. Keep the list of the two (or more) activities in your pocket or in a reminder app on your phone.
3. Plan to do the activities daily. As with every suggestion in this book, if you don't do them every day, don't get down on yourself; just commit to do them the next day.
4. After some time, add activities to the list, so you have a menu to choose from. Change them up, so you do something different for a day or two.

Acting from the outside in is such a key component to living well with depression that it is reiterated numerous times throughout this book. Use it often and in different situations. Over time and with practice, this effort will come more intuitively. In fact, there is emerging neuroscience data that activity may affect our brains positively and improve our ability to experience pleasure or satisfaction.

"I'm so irritable that I just lash out at everyone."

Keep in mind that the problem is not being irritable; the problem is that you lash out or act according to the action urge in the emotional response. You don't need to fear your feelings. Here are some straightforward emotion regulation strategies that can help. You only need willingness, not great skill, to do them.

COUNT TO TEN

Believe it or not, counting to 10 might work. When you're feeling very irritable, counting gives you a little time to stop and think before acting on impulse. You may actually need to count to 100. The number is completely irrelevant. What's important is to stop, step back (metaphorically or literally), and think before you respond. There isn't anything wrong with feeling irritable and wanting to lash out, it's only problematic to actually lash out.

BREATHE

Use the power of breathing. Your breathing does more than just supply your body with oxygen and clear out toxins. You can slow your breathing and reduce physiological responses to high emotional arousal. Try this simple breathing exercise:

1. Sit comfortably and inhale through your nose, counting slowly to four.
2. Hold your breath for another slow count of four.
3. Now exhale through your mouth, slowly, to a count of four.
4. Bring your attention to your breathing, to the feeling of the cool air coming in through your nostrils.
5. Notice any tension in your chest as you hold your breath; then release it as you exhale. Do this for several minutes, if you can; if you're particularly harried with chores, children, or coworkers, even doing this quietly for 15 to 20 seconds can help.

BE ASSERTIVE, NOT AGGRESSIVE

You may get more irritable when you feel that you are not getting your needs met, or that others aren't properly caring for you. It's your right to ask for what you need and want. However, for some people, it can be difficult to ask; for some, only the heat of anger or irritability gives them the power to state their needs.

When you are angry, your needs may be expressed aggressively, creating more problems over time. Experts on assertiveness training suggest that you consider asking for what will *effectively* get you what you need. Imagine being behind a car that doesn't move forward after the streetlight turns green. You can tap your horn or lay on the horn for a solid 30 seconds. Which ask is likely to be more effective at getting you what you need? Tapping lets the driver in front know they need to get moving; laying on the horn lets them know you're fed up with them, which will likely result in them making a rude gesture out of their window, making you even angrier.

So, do what the assertiveness experts call the "minimally effective response"—just enough to get your needs met, and not so much that it releases all your anger or frustration or causes more.

"My sadness and misery spill into every area of my life."

When you feel overwhelmed, it's hard to take your attention off the sadness and misery. It hurts, and when something hurts, you tend to it. This makes perfect sense. If you were to accidentally hit your thumb with a hammer while hanging a picture, you might put it in your mouth, or grab it with your other hand, or quickly get some ice. You tend to what hurts you. But you wouldn't keep your thumb packed in ice for an entire day.

Focusing on your sadness is understandable, but following the urge to indulge it, to tell everyone about it, to approach every situation with a sad face and hope for empathy from others may backfire, and become overwhelming for those around you as well. Don't ignore your depression, but don't dwell on it either.

BE AN ACTIVE LISTENER

A simple solution to dwelling on your misery—which doesn't require that you deny it—is to ask others about themselves. Listen to what they have to say. Resist the urge to jump into your story as soon as they finish a sentence. Sharing space for someone else to express themselves can allow for a mutual exchange of caring. It can be like having only a small bowl of food between two people; eating all of it yourself can satisfy your hunger, but sharing it can keep both people alive.

TAKE A RISK

If your tendency is to keep your feelings to yourself, share something with somebody you trust. Let down the "I've got it all together" facade.

Telling others about your inner life, even about an emotional struggle, may make you more approachable. It won't open the floodgates of your emotions, nor will it likely open floodgates from others. You don't need to fear some dreaded forced group hug. Just share something that allows others to get to know you better.

Living Well

- Making peace with and allowing our emotions is the wisest, most skillful thing we can do to keep ourselves in good mental shape.
- We also can regulate our emotions, so we don't become overwhelmed by them, by remembering the ARC of emotions: Antecedent, Response, and Consequence.
- Taking a thoughtful approach to emotional expression can be helpful in regulating irritability or overwhelming sadness, and getting your needs met.

2

behaviors

BE PROACTIVE

It's counterintuitive, but when you're feeling overwhelmed, bogged down, unable to get out of the pit of feeling bad, taking action is the best medicine. Physical therapists like to say, "Motion is lotion," and this is true for mental health as well. Being active and engaged—even knitting qualifies!—has been shown to improve mood and reduce anxiety.

Is Behavior a Choice?

As we discussed in Chapter 1, in the ARC of emotion, the emotional response (the "R") consists of sensations, feelings, thoughts, and behaviors. We often fail to recognize that much of our behavior is automatic. It's a response to the events of our day, and like our thoughts and beliefs, it's subject to the conditioning that has occurred throughout our lives. For instance, if you hear a bump in the middle of the night, you might awaken with a start and hide under your blankets; nudge your spouse to see what's happening; or grab a bat and go look for yourself. While some of your reaction has a biological or temperamental aspect, it's also the result of how you've been conditioned. If you've had trauma when you were young, you may feel safer under the blankets. If you've experienced success at taking charge or have been taught that you need to be brave, you may be the one to pick up the bat.

So, yes, behavior is also a choice. When you're sad, you may indeed choose to retreat from loved ones. To a great extent, however, those choices are based on what you have experienced in the past. If retreat has resulted in relief, you will do that. When you reach out to others and they sympathize, you will be more likely to reach out in the future. Ironically, our behaviors don't always provide the results we desire. Have you ever thought that giving someone a "piece of your mind" would feel good and teach them a lesson, only to find that they reacted with anger and you felt ashamed that you harmed a relationship?

As discussed in Chapter 1, Barlow and colleagues, who coined the acronym ARC, refer to the behavioral part of an emotional response as an action urge. The urge is what is often out of our awareness, and automatic; following through to *act* on the urge is usually where choice comes in. Since we take so many actions without really being aware, it can be very helpful to take time to understand how your behaviors serve you. We tend to not consider the consequences of the small actions we take every day.

Why Do We Try to Escape or Avoid Our Feelings?

It's no surprise that we are strongly conditioned to do things that help us avoid pain. Your attempts to escape from pain, the emotional numbing, and the disengagement from activities that once gave you pleasure makes sense.

In Chapter 1, you learned ways to practice having a different relationship with your feelings. You can also gain strategies that lead to a different relationship with automatic behaviors and responses to action urges. Psychologists have several names for this process, including *functional analysis* and *using opposite action*. Here, we call it *acting from the outside in*, as discussed in Chapter 1, and the ABCs.

The ABCs

The ABCs stand for:

- **A:** *Antecedent,* or what comes before an event occurs
- **B:** *Behavior* that you take
- **C:** *Consequence* of the action (behavior) taken

It's easy to understand the ABCs when you reflect on situations in which the consequences were either really bad or really good. For example, if you were rushing in your kitchen while baking a casserole and reached for the hot dish from the oven with your bare hands, only to have burned fingers, you would recognize the consequence of rushing and likely not forget to get a potholder prior to opening the oven door in the future. Alternatively, if you had a very successful karaoke night performance, you would easily make the connection between singing at karaoke and receiving resounding applause. That would stand out as a really good consequence, and you'd be likely to continue going to karaoke night. Those situations are memorable. You realized the consequence was something you don't want to happen again, and you told yourself, "I'll never do that again." Or, on the opposite side, you may have thought, "More please!" when your behavior resulted in getting you something wonderful.

But there are daily consequences, little things, that influence our moods that we don't really think about. In fact, they not only get overlooked by ourselves, they get overlooked by others, sometimes even by mental health providers. And yet, it's the everyday actions we take, over and over, day after day, without awareness, that contribute to our mood state far more often than big events.

Over the years, I have consulted with therapists doing research on behavioral activation (BA) as a treatment for depression and anxiety. I've concluded from these studies that recognizing the consequences of daily activities is a key to living well. And the simple attention to the ABCs helped some participants to act more consistently with their values and to engage in meaningful activities—two pathways to a fulfilling, satisfying life.[1,2]

Nearly all of the strategies offered in this chapter call on some aspect of the ABCs. As you read about what you can do differently in common daily scenarios, think about how you're using the ABCs as a lens to help you become more aware of automatic behaviors, and take mindful actions that support your well-being.

Acting from the Outside In

When you're depressed, you act in the best way that you can to feel better. The problem is that when your goal is to escape from the feelings (or lack of feeling) associated with depression, you can act in ways that pull you away from your true values. When you begin to recognize that the outcome of your behavior (the *consequence* in the ABCs) is to escape or avoid a negative emotional experience, you have a clue that you may be acting from the "inside out." You are being controlled by your feelings. This is natural, we all do it; recognizing it is not an invitation to self-blame! From the perspective of behavioral psychologists, when behavior is controlled by its consequences, all behavior makes sense.

Acting from the outside in allows you to take steps toward what's meaningful, even if it doesn't give you an emotional sensation of pleasure or enjoyment. You need to keep acting from the outside until it gets *in*—until there is enjoyment or until you're living in a more consistent way with what you value, even if you still feel depressed. It's unrealistic to think that you can just white-knuckle your way through rough times. By acting in a way consistent with your values and goals, you can experience tiny successes at achieving what you set out to do, even very small things.

For instance, I don't always feel like sitting down to write, and writing doesn't always come easily to me. But I believe this book is important, and writing about BA and other ways to help people through depression is consistent with my values. However, many other things pull at me. So, I play with the dog or binge on a television series—I act from the inside out, from what I feel like doing. When I write even one paragraph, however, it moves me toward a goal—I'm acting from the outside in, from my plan. Yes, the writing is a struggle, but I do it anyway. Over time, I get more words on the page, and the ideas slowly begin to flow, and it's less of a struggle. The action has changed the feeling, and motivation to write has followed the action of writing.

Acting As If

Acting as if is a scripted technique that can slowly provide some relief from deep misery. We touched on this concept briefly in Chapter 1. The main idea is to use your power of choice to act in a way that will serve several purposes. With acting as if, you might simply be able to get through a difficult moment, or you may actually end up with a shift in your mood. Acting as if allows you to hold the feeling you have, but to define what needs to be done in ways that follow values-driven behaviors. Admittedly, it will feel like "going through the motions" at first. However, you can think of outside in as representing the direction, with the outcome being that your actions will, over time, change your mood.

Let's take a few moments to play around with the idea of acting as if. The objective is to act, or to be an actor. In method acting, actors immerse themselves in the roles of the characters they are playing. They rely on sensation memories from their own lives to bring up emotions naturally to give a realistic performance. They aren't faking, but they are indeed playing a role. In the same way, we need to be ourselves, but act from a different mood, doing things differently than our current feelings may seem to dictate. So, let's give acting as if a try:

- **What parts of the activity are you going to do?** Identify a task that you do by rote, perhaps getting dressed in the morning. Break it down. You may start with choosing the pieces of your outfit. Then you might need to match accessories, like a belt, so pick out those too. Then you might put on your trousers one leg at a time. Then you'll put on the other pieces. The point is that activities that we do daily become automatic, and to act as if, we need to think about the various parts of even the most rote activities.
- **What would your body be doing if you were feeling sad?** Turn on a piece of music that is evocative for you and that can

sometimes make you feel sad. Sit in a chair with your shoulders down, feet stretched out in front of you, and just let yourself slump down. Put your head down as if your neck can't even hold the weight. Frown. Perhaps close, or mostly close your eyes. If your eyes are open, just stare at a spot on the floor until your vision loses focus. How do you feel? I presume you feel a little blue. While listening to this music, you have just acted as if you were sad and blue, and it may have evoked that feeling. It may have been easy for you to evoke that feeling if you have been depressed of late. This sets up the next step: acting as if you are not blue.

• **What would your body be doing if you were feeling . . . different?** Keep the same music playing and sit up straight in your chair. Lift your head and either look forward or turn from side to side. Open your eyes and lift your eyebrows slightly. Don't exaggerate, but do elevate them a little. If you're near a window, look outside and find shimmering leaves, a passerby, or cars moving along. If you aren't near a window, just look around the room. Raise the corners of your mouth, again just slightly. You don't have to put on a big smile (that would be faking and possibly a little creepy). Keep your shoulders high.

Now, how do you feel? At this point, I assume you might feel a little different, maybe a little silly, which is just fine. But I presume you don't feel the pull of the gloom from the sad music as much as you did when you were slumped in the chair with your body and muscles telling you that what you are experiencing is misery. The point is that simply changing your body posture can change how you feel. This is likely why there is evidence to suggest that injections of Botox can improve depression. Presumably this is because Botox does things like lift the eyebrows as it tightens the skin, a facial movement we associate with feeling engaged and upbeat. You can act as if for any feeling—whether it's happy, confident, brave, or anything else.

• **How would you talk to others?** Finally, you may notice that when you're depressed you tend to speak in monotone and sometimes mumble. Speak up. Take a deep breath from your belly to give your voice some power. Articulate your words. Imagine someone in the back of a large auditorium who needs to hear you without a microphone. You don't need to shout, but just speak clearly, as if you were a confident public speaker. You can also imagine a script for an actor written to provide a certain mood. Does the script for someone who is not depressed include talking only about struggles, hurts, indignities? Probably not. The script is probably also not all about marvelously fun and cheerful things with sugary platitudes about how wonderful the world is. A realistic script would evoke what people normally talk about. Tell someone you like a particular color they are wearing, or make a statement about the weather, or about something unusual that you notice. Realistic scripts may be more neutral than positive, and that is fine. You don't need to fake being upbeat, just act as if you aren't sad, anxious, angry, or whatever emotion is strong and likely to get you stuck acting from the inside out.

Silas's Story

Like me, Silas had worked throughout his professional life as a therapist helping clients living with depression and anxiety. Also like me, he could empathize but had never felt the depth of depression himself. Then he had a a major medical event that required surgery. He woke up in the recovery room after having a traumatic experience with only a shadow memory of being hoisted in a sling and put to bed while in great pain. Lying in his bed, he felt utter despair. There was no pain in his body, there were no thoughts of a bleak future, there was just trauma, and deep gloom that left him wanting nothing but to be dead. There were no feelings to flee; there was, in his words, "just nothing but utter hopelessness." Silas was not a man who had ever considered taking his life, but at that moment all he yearned for was to cease to exist.

Silas lay in this state for several days. The nursing staff urged him to get out of bed, to stand up. He didn't care; it meant nothing to him. Then he awoke one morning, as he described it, "with Christopher in my head." He had been discussing behavioral activation with me for many years, so he knew what to do. He told himself to get up and walk; he did a half lap around the nurses' station, just as the nurses had been telling him to for days. He acted from the outside in. He followed what was consistent with a goal of healing, although at that moment he had no motivation to heal. He knew that the despair was pulling him deeper and that he had a choice to let it continue to pull him down or do what he and I had talked about, had helped others to do, and knew was difficult but necessary: He took that first small step.

Changing Your Relationship to Your Actions

Below are some common statements that I've heard over many years of working with people who live with depression. Some have felt the kind of despair described by my friend Silas. For them, this was the state of their lives, and it was exhausting, but they didn't care enough to do much about it—although coming to therapy was a step in the right direction. When you have similar feelings and taking action feels impossible, try some of the techniques here.

> *"When I feel blue, I don't want to do anything but scroll through my phone."*

Depression can be a state of inertia. The action urge is to do nothing at all. Engaging in a mindless activity like aimlessly scrolling through your phone—or even just sitting and staring at nothing—can have a strong pull. As an antidote, you don't need to feel motivated, you don't need to care, you just need to act.

PLAN A GO-TO ACTIVITY AHEAD OF TIME

Planning activities in advance is a very helpful solution. The key is to do this when you're not in a state of inertia. Then, when you're feeling stuck, you don't have to think about what to do, you've practiced ahead of time. When you haven't been motivated to do anything for some time, the place to start is with some very simple activities that you can decide to do and that will be successful.

1. Use an activity log to schedule one activity over the next week.
2. Schedule things that bring you a sense of pleasure, are values-

guided, or just get you moving, such as walking into a different room and stretching your arms toward the ceiling.

3. Take the first step. A second is likely to follow. Keep in mind that if you had broken your leg, you would not start rehabilitation by jogging on a treadmill; rather, you'd probably start with a few very simple knee-bend exercises. Whatever your equivalent of a knee bend is, start there. Once you've done that, you will have acted on a plan—and that is success.

KEEP AN ACTIVITY–MOOD CHART

Going back to the ABCs, one consequence (C) of behavior (B) that you can begin to notice is your mood. By paying attention, you can gain a clearer understanding of how your behaviors relate to, and even shape, your mood. You can also begin to see how closely your life now aligns with the kind of life you value.

Start by completing an Activity–Mood Chart on the facing page. You may use the one provided (extra charts may be downloaded from *www.guilford.com/martell3-materials*). Write down what you were doing in hourly increments. Include the activity, and with whom you did it. Also write your predominant feeling during that hour of the day.

If pausing to write down every hour of the day feels overwhelming, break the day into four-hour chunks, as in the shaded area. Then write at least three times a day: morning, midday, and evening. Recall the previous three or four hours and note what you were doing and how you were feeling. The more often you can track your hours, the more data you will gather. But writing just three or four times a day is better than nothing.

When you keep a log of your activities, you might be surprised to see how much your moods change during the day and how related they are to what you're doing. You might also discover that you have consistent patterns you hadn't noticed before.

"Everything feels tedious."

Life can become routine for anyone. Routines are good for us, and can be comforting—but when routine becomes boring, or when

ACTIVITY–MOOD CHART

Time	Activity (what and with whom)	Feeling
12 A.M.		
1 A.M.		
2 A.M.		
3 A.M.		
4 A.M.		
5 A.M.		
6 A.M.		
7 A.M.		
8 A.M.		
9 A.M.		
10 A.M.		
11 A.M.		
12 P.M.		
1 P.M.		
2 P.M.		
3 P.M.		
4 P.M.		
5 P.M.		
6 P.M.		
7 P.M.		
8 P.M.		
9 P.M.		
10 P.M.		
11 P.M.		

depression steals your interest in everyday activities, it can become difficult to keep moving forward. Starting small, you can add some new activities to your schedule that can shift your routine.

You might be thinking, "But everything is tedious! What's the point?" The point is that when you're in a rut, small changes to your routine can, over time, make a difference.

Sometimes there are necessary tasks that you simply can't find the motivation for, because they seem boring. Boredom is an indication that you're not fully engaging in life; getting out of that avoidance trap and doing the task may be a good first step. Here is one way to do that:

LIST A SERIES OF SMALL STEPS

1. Make a plan for taking small steps.
2. Rate how difficult each step can be.
3. Decide in advance whether you will start with one or two of the steps.
4. Decide in advance whether you'll do the hardest or the easiest task first.

Doing the hardest task first might give you a sense of accomplishment and then make all of the following steps seem much easier. Doing the easiest task first can get you started and earn you an initial success—and might be the only way you can do anything at all.

ENHANCE THE ACTIVITY

You've probably heard of "enhanced" water—which is really plain old water with some extra minerals or flavoring, so it's ostensibly more enjoyable. Bring this approach to tedious activities. For instance, consider acting as if you were enjoying the activity, or competent at it. Or add something pleasurable, like your favorite music playing in the background. If the task can be done in public, take it to a park or coffee shop. Invite a friend to join you with something they need to get done. This may sound strange, but we join with others for book clubs and knitting circles—why not ask someone to join you in a "let's get one project done" afternoon?

"Doing anything seems overwhelming."

This is extremely common when you're depressed. Many life situations are genuinely overwhelming. Financial concerns, illness, interpersonal problems, employment troubles, or housing issues all can overwhelm. The bar for what feels overwhelming gets lower when you're depressed. Take the example of cleaning a sink and counters full of dirty dishes. You might start by simply putting greasy pans in dishwater to soak. Ah, but now that they've soaked, you might as well just wash them. And now that the dishwater is dirty, how about draining it? But then you've got an empty sink—may as well add clean, hot dishwater so you can wash glasses . . . and then silverware.

Wait! This all seems very practical, but what if it still winds up being overwhelming? If you succeed with step one, there is nothing wrong with doing the other steps. But—and here's the takeaway—*it can be unhelpful to think that every time you start something you need to do it all.* Because if you can't allow yourself to stop at step one or two, every task and every situation will feel big and continue to overwhelm you.

Here's an old saying: "How do you eat an elephant? One bite at a time." With apologies to our pachyderm friends, there is wisdom here: What initially seems impossible only gets done in incremental steps.

BREAK THINGS DOWN

1. Set the goal of doing just parts of the task.
2. Then, break the task down into five or six small steps.
3. Break down those steps into even smaller steps.
4. Remember, your goal is not to complete the entire task, but to start with just one or two steps and allow yourself to stop there. (If you continue, that's okay, but the point here is to reduce overwhelm with fewer steps, not maintain overwhelm by doing it all.)
5. Make a plan for each of the future steps, and schedule times to do them.

PRACTICE DOING ONE THING MINDFULLY

Another way to manage tasks that are tedious or overwhelming is to do a small task mindfully. This means focusing your attention on all aspects of the task. Notice what you see, smell, feel, and hear. Keep bringing your attention back to those things when your mind wanders. Take your time. The goal is not completion—the goal is mindful attention.

You might be doing something as simple as making the bed. Notice the feeling of the air rushing through when you fluff the sheets. Inhale the scent. Notice the difference in the feel of the sheet and the bedspread . . . the thickness and textures. Listen attentively to the sounds of the fabrics as you arrange them. Smooth out wrinkles. Doing this mundane task mindfully may engage you in a way you haven't experienced before, and offer a break from hectic demands. You may turn something routine—something you usually just get out of the way on autopilot—into a moment that feels fresh.

"I'm busy all the time. How can I do more?"

You might think that doing a task mindfully is just a waste of time. Or that activation sounds dreadful because you already have too much to do. If you've had those thoughts, you are not alone. Depressed people don't always just sit around staring at walls. You may be too busy, have too many demands, and work all the time, yet you're still depressed. A few suggestions can help if this is your situation.

SET PRIORITIES

We can get pulled into doing things that don't make us happy or provide the fulfillment we expected. This is when it's worth pausing to ask whether what keeps us so busy is actually consistent with our values. Work may be extremely demanding, or you may have a lot to do to keep your children in school and fed. Regardless of your situation, you need to prioritize the things that need to be done.

Airplane safety instructions tell us to put on our own oxygen mask before helping others. That is a set priority. So, you might start there. What do you need to do to keep yourself healthy enough to actually complete your tasks? Your own physical and mental health may need to be your first priority. This might mean giving up some of your other responsibilities. You set priorities by asking what is consistent with your values.

EVALUATE THE CONSEQUENCES OF YOUR BEHAVIOR

You can use the ABCs from earlier in this chapter to look at the consequences of your behavior. Doing so can help you gain insight into how closely you're living in accordance with your values. Let's look at one example:

- **A:** *Antecedent:* Bills come in the mail.
- **B:** *Behavior:* I stack the bills in a pile to pay later.
- **C:** *Consequence:* I feel immediate relief that I don't have to stop and handle them right away, and I turn my attention to preparing a meal . . . but I do feel some guilt because they're important . . . and sometimes I don't pay the bills for a month or two, and then I have to pay late fees.

Is the consequence in accordance with this person's values? Immediately yes, if this person values family bonding and prioritizes dinner with loved ones over sitting down to pay bills. But if bills go unpaid too long, late fees apply, and this conflicts with this person's value of fiscal responsibility. Looking at the ABCs, this person might conclude stacking bills is fine—but only for a week or two.

Choose several tasks in your life, apply the ABCs, and identify whether adjustments are needed so that you're acting in accordance with your values.

"I don't even want to get out of bed in the morning!"

All of the suggestions in this book so far may simply feel like too much. You may have tried many things and still live with depression. You may feel numb. I understand! That is why the activities in this book are designed to help you develop the habit of living according to a plan rather than a mood or feeling. The kind of activity is less important than the decision to take small steps toward breaking the grip of the mood.

START WITH YOUR FEET ON THE FLOOR

Your bed may feel like a place of safety; you pull the covers over your head and avoid facing the day. Or you may be having thoughts like, "I'm letting everyone down," "I'm lazy and useless," and on and on. Let those thought bubbles float away for now. Concentrate on just one goal, one demand: Put your feet on the floor.

1. Set an alarm for any time of the day that you think is realistic. No judgment. Could be 7 A.M. or 1 P.M.
2. When that alarm rings, sit up, swing your body around, and place your feet on the floor.
3. Stay sitting up for at least one to five minutes.
4. Congratulate yourself because you have met your goal!

Do this every day. Whatever else you may end up doing that day is a bonus. If you do nothing else, that's okay, because, for now, you have met the goal. You've broken the habit of drowning in a mood and surfaced for some fresh air for a few seconds.

PLAN SIMPLE MORNING ACTIVITIES

You won't be living well if you only put your feet on the floor for an extended period of time, though. It will be important to begin engaging in life. Start small. Go from sitting to standing. From standing to walking, and so forth. Simple morning routines can be accomplished whether you are rich or poor, whether you are physically able to do them on your own or need some assistance. Here is a list of things to consider doing. Start with one or two and add more as you go:

- Open the blinds
- Splash water on your face

- Wash your face thoroughly
- Get a drink of water
- Fix a cup of coffee or tea
- Eat a banana or a bowl of cereal
- Comb or brush your hair
- Shave if you need to
- Take a shower

Over time, you will be out of your bed, getting ready in the morning and doing simple things to face the day. Even in the darkest times, you can do something very small. Have empathy for yourself. Even in deep suffering, take charge of something small that moves you toward living well.

Living Well

- You can change how you feel by changing what you do.
- You can even change how things work in your brain by adjusting your actions and thoughts.
- You can become and stay engaged in your life, which will keep your depression manageable.
- It makes perfect sense to disengage when you're depressed. But this disengagement reinforces itself like a habit. Fortunately, you can break the habit by taking small steps to act according to what you value and the goals you set, and not according to the mood that's pulling you down.

3

thoughts

THINK FLEXIBLY

Our thoughts are tricky! They're not always accurate, they can prolong our emotional state, and sometimes we overidentify with them. All of us have opinions—about the world, about others, about ourselves—and frequently those opinions are wrong or irrelevant. Guess what? We don't have to believe everything we think. We also don't need to live in a world of our own making with thoughts that pull our attention too much inward.

When you hurt, you tend to that pain. This is true if you are stung by a bee and move your hand to swat it away, and it's true when your mood is low and your attention becomes focused on how bad you feel. It's natural to do this; it makes total sense. However, too much focus on emotional pain can also be problematic, as depressive thoughts have a rigid and negative nature. Depressive thoughts make you unusually hard on yourself, prone to misinterpreting the motivations of others. They don't make the future look bright. The pull of these thoughts disengages you from life, as if you're looking only at your feet and cannot see the horizon or what else is around you. It makes sense, keeping with this metaphor, that if you're feeling fragile you need to watch carefully where you walk. But when you're feeling depressed and focusing on it, your brain brings your full attention to your low mood.

In other words, your thought process, the kinds of thoughts you have, and your conditioning throughout life all play a role in linking your thoughts to feelings. Your thoughts are powerful! You may not be able to move mountains with your thoughts, but you can make yourself feel worse by the thoughts you have. Fortunately, this phenomenon works in the other direction. You can also make yourself feel better by thinking differently. This chapter explores how to do that. First, though, let's learn more about our thoughts and our tendencies when it comes to thinking.

What Is Flexible Thinking?

Your thinking can become *rigid* when a particular mood dominates. For example, when depression takes over, much of your thinking may turn to the hopelessness of it all. Similarly, anxiety can lead to rigid thoughts about the dangers around you, and anger can keep you fully believing that people are truly as nasty as you imagine. The rigidity is also the mood pulling you in.

Have you ever started your day on the wrong foot? Maybe you got up in the morning, burned your breakfast, stubbed your toe, and jumped in a shower only to find the water is cold—and you think, "This day is going to suck!" You might then start your commute and tell yourself all of the traffic is getting in your way, the subway is full of jerks, and now the day is ruined. You are then stuck in the belief that "Everything is horrible." When you judge yourself, get stuck in absolutes, and don't take a moment to consider that all may not be as hopeless as you think, it's like staring straight ahead and forgetting that there are things to see on either side and behind you.

To offset this, consider the possibility that other things may be true. The ability to consider alternatives is known as *flexible thinking.* You cannot possibly have all of the information about yourself or the world, so consider alternatives to your thoughts, developing flexibility. For example, the "maniac" who just cut you off on the freeway may be rushing home to a sick child. Or, referring back to the bad-morning example, the traffic and subway commuters might be just as they always are. Yet, when you believe your self-talk about the day being ruined, nothing else seems to go right.

Generally, just as movement is important for physical health, flexibility in thinking is important for mental health. Such flexibility is not the same as being open-minded, although that may be part of it for a number of people. Flexible thinking is more about finding ways of thinking that result in greater contentment and hope. It allows us to navigate a variety of nuanced situations without getting stuck. The second half of this chapter is chock-full of ways to practice flexible thinking.

Why Are Some Thoughts Emotional?

Some therapists look at thoughts as words that have taken on the emotional properties that they are intended to represent. It's similar to how the word "elephant" brings up a picture in your head of a large, gray pachyderm. There's a figurative correlation. But now imagine that the word "elephant" could also make you nearly stop breathing, from the thought of a heavy giant sitting on your chest. That's a physical correlation. Now imagine that the word "elephant" brought the feeling of loss—a gargantuan feeling of deep and heavy loss every time you think the word "elephant."

Researchers and therapists who work from this perspective would say that you are *fused* with your thoughts when the emotion or your identity is commingled with the thought. It's like when you put sugar in water; you have two different substances that, when blended and stirred together, seem to be just one. If you boil away the water, it will turn to steam, and you'll be left again with the sugar. Thankfully, you don't need to boil your thoughts to *defuse* from them. When you defuse from your thoughts (see tip later in this chapter), certain words won't hold as much emotional power over you.

Do Our Moods Color Our Mind?

Two famous psychotherapists, Aaron T. Beck and Albert Ellis, revolutionized the field of psychology when they observed that their patients' expressed beliefs were associated with their emotional distress. Beck worked with depressed patients and noticed that depressed patients shared similar thought patterns, distinct from those of non-depressed people.

You likely recognize yourself in this. When depressed, perceptions of the world around you, of other people, and of yourself become particularly negative. Beck and Ellis proposed that unhelpful thoughts and beliefs affect our moods in ways that contribute to poor mental health. They proposed that a way to reverse this pattern is to help people change their thoughts; later, Christine Padesky and Dennis Greenberger referred to that theory in the title of their famous self-help book, *Mind Over Mood.*

As you read this chapter, consider whether your thoughts reflect the reality of the world around you, or whether they are predominantly colored by your mood. If you're looking at the world through gray-colored glasses, everything can seem dull, boring, hopeless. Yet, that is not a true reflection of your environment or your life. When you focus on everything being negative, and miss out on the positives, that imbalance will pull you into depression.

Let's look at this from another perspective. In the Western world, where we put so much emphasis on individualism, we think highly of ourselves and our self-determination. All of that is great, but we can forget that we are products of our environment. If you've been mistreated by others, either when you were young or at present, it stands to reason that you may begin to think that you deserve it. Don't bad things happen to bad people? Well, yes and no. The reality is that bad things happen to people *and* also good things happen.

Good things can happen to good people, and depression can still loom. A privileged, happy world can become colorless and bleak. This is also not your fault. You can't always control your thoughts and feelings, although you can choose how you act on them.

In essence, it's healthy when you can see yourself, the world around you, and other people in your life in a balanced way. To do this, it's helpful to think critically about your own thinking. Evaluating your thoughts requires that you open yourself to the possibility that your beliefs are not 100 percent correct.

I'm not implying that some of your thoughts are "bad" or that you're out of touch with reality; I'm saying that you can and should consider other possibilities, as part of flexible thinking. Look for evidence that your thoughts may not reflect *all* of your reality. You'll have plenty of evidence of negative thoughts, since that is where a blue mood has pulled your focus. You must work a little harder to find evidence of positive thoughts, or even neutral ones. We'll dive into this more in Part Two of the book, so this chapter is a warm-up.

How Do Our Beliefs Tell Stories?

One of the most difficult things that happens when we're depressed is that our thoughts can turn dark or negative toward ourselves, others, and the future. This is when our *core beliefs* start to play in our heads.[1] Overlearned and well-practiced throughout our lives, they are the negative stories we repeatedly tell ourselves and deeply believe. They are absolutes like "I am unlovable," "People are unkind," and "The world is terrible." The core beliefs in your mind can vary and will be unique to you, but they feel as if they're true. They can be so ingrained that you feel it "in your skin," so to speak.

Related to core beliefs are *schemas,* which are the overarching attitudes, beliefs, and perceptions we have of ourselves. They are often made up of several core beliefs and tend to be broader. You developed schemas when you were growing up. You likely weren't aware of their presence then, or now, but they influence how you are in the world.

Psychologist Jeffrey Young identified a number of schemas and their impact. Young also calls schemas *life traps;* here are a few common ones:[2]

- **Vulnerability,** in which we see the world as dangerous and ourselves as unable to meet the challenges of life
- **Abandonment,** or a belief that others will leave us and we can't rely on them
- **Defectiveness,** or the belief that we're somehow flawed or broken
- **Subjugation,** or a pattern of putting others before ourselves to the point where we're always in second place

These schemas are so absolute that they can influence our responses to everyday situations in unhelpful ways. They dictate the rules that we live by.

For example, if you have an abandonment schema, you may have a core belief that you are unlovable. When you only see through the gray-colored glasses of that schema, you attend to information that supports those beliefs. Everywhere you look, you see evidence that seems to prove the belief true. Every time you do something wrong or miss the mark, you see it as more evidence. Likewise, when you do something right, you discount it. Since that outcome doesn't fit your belief and isn't part of the story you tell yourself, you dismiss it. Even when you feel momentarily proud of yourself, you likely find a believable reason that your accomplishment was not all that good.

Wholeheartedly believing your core belief is like listening to a choir but only being able to hear the bass section. You will think that the song is always low, and you'll hear that full bass note proving that songs are only made for deep voices. When you hear a lovely melody from a soprano, it will sound odd. You may enjoy it for a minute, but then write it off as being someone singing wrong notes. Imagine what all music would sound like if this were your interpretation of it. You might even be called "tonally challenged" because you weren't hearing the actual, true notes.

Every one of us can be tonally challenged about ourselves. There are rational reasons for this. A main reason is that our beliefs are often met with "proof" from others. For example, if you had parents or teachers repeatedly tell you "I figured you'd fail" when you did poorly on a test, you might believe you are incapable or stupid. Even if you achieve some success, you might hear "Don't get too pleased with yourself; you know you usually don't do well" from someone else or even yourself.

It's as if our negative core beliefs are like terry cloth sweaters, and the proof of it like balls of Velcro that stick. Our positive experiences are like ping-pong balls that tap us but then bounce off. The truth is, you aren't stuck in your story, even when it feels that way. We hear about people "reinventing" themselves all the time. You can do that too, even if it's reinventing your understanding of yourself. In fact, Young cowrote the self-help book *Reinventing Your Life,* which offers strategies for specifically addressing schemas.

All of us have things that we would like to change about ourselves. You likely have some idea of what you want to change. Or, because of the depression, you may have lost sight of the things about yourself that are great just the way they are. You can rediscover yourself. You need not be held hostage by the story you have come to believe over the years.

Can't We Just Make Our Thoughts Go Away?

Usually, wanting our thoughts to stop running through our brain only keeps them going. Wishing a thought to go away, or trying to avoid emotions that we experience as negative, keeps us stuck—embroiled in a battle with ourselves.

This is where acceptance and commitment therapy (ACT) is helpful. It encourages us to change the context of our thinking, or to shift our relationship to our thoughts. Basically, we acknowledge the thought but refrain from responding automatically to it. Cognitive therapists have a similar approach, objectively evaluating the content of our thoughts.

Our busy brain is always telling a story. Nope, we can't stop our thoughts from flowing, but we can develop the practice of *defusing* (ACT) from our thoughts. Simply put, this strategy is about breaking free of the conditioned emotional connection to thoughts and looking at a thought as a thing that is neither factual, nor part of you. Put another way, a thought is merely an interpretation that makes sense given our personal histories, but it's not necessarily true. You're invited to try this strategy in the section "Say, 'I'm Having the Thought That . . .' " below.

MONITOR YOUR THOUGHTS

There's some irony in suggesting that you track your moods and thoughts. Here's the challenge: It's helpful to know what's going through your mind when your moods change, but it's not helpful to fixate on your thoughts and moods. One solution is to do just enough self-monitoring to see the patterns of your thinking that may bring you low or keep you feeling blue, then move on. This, then, is step one: becoming aware of how your thoughts and moods are connected, so you can progress to the important work of thinking differently.

To monitor your reactions to events, grab a notebook or a sheet of paper and create two columns. Write down the following:

1. The situation that occurred, in the left column
2. The thought that came to mind, in the right column

It doesn't need to be more complicated than that. Do this as often as you can for a full week. If you have more than one thought per situation, write them all down. Your list might look like this:

Situation	Thought
Got honked at	I am a bad driver
Misplaced keys	I am an idiot

Once you've collected a week's worth of self-monitoring data, see if your thoughts tend to skew toward the negative or if they may be reflecting a sad or angry mood. Use them as clues to what you may deeply believe about yourself, others, or the world. Notice whether they might be confirming a schema or core belief that you weren't even aware of.

With your self-monitoring data in hand, it's also a good time to enlist a trusted person as a reality check. You can ask them if they think they might have the same reaction to the situations you've listed.

Changing Your Relationship to Your Thoughts

Our busy brains are always interpreting things that are happening to us. As we've discussed, many of those thoughts can be negative and believable, even when not true. In the rest of this chapter, we'll look at common thoughts that represent the types of "distortions" described by Beck and others. As a cognitive-behavioral psychologist, I've heard many variations of these thoughts, and as a human being, I've thought many of them as well.

You can change the thoughts that make you unhappy. Just as you've done with emotions, you do this by accepting your tendencies to think in particular ways and being open to relating to them differently. This work begins with identifying those thoughts.

"My life is terrible."

A thought like this is an *overgeneralization,* or a conclusion that is more sweeping than is justified. In reality, there are very few people for whom every minute of every day is terrible. People often have this kind of thought when they are in a difficult, perhaps even devastating, situation. However, the description is usually not reflective of your whole life. When you overgeneralize, it's helpful to do the following:

1. Actively consider other options. Is it possible that you're overstating the facts?
2. Look for evidence that disproves the rule (see next strategy). If there is one good thing in your life, it isn't all terrible.
3. Restate the belief in a less absolutist way. Then, consider if the revised description is actually more accurate, for example, "I'm having a rough day [or week, month, year], but my life has had ups as well as downs."
4. Assess if you feel a change in your mood when you consider alternatives to the belief.

LOOK FOR EVIDENCE

If you have a particularly unflattering opinion of yourself, or beliefs that the world is malevolent, it's not difficult to find evidence that supports your view. But you're also ignoring information that doesn't fit your *self-concept* or beliefs about the world. What you're experiencing as your reality is only part of the actual picture. So, consider what you might be missing.

What are the ping-pong balls that bounce off rather than stick to your core belief sweater? What are the facts of your situation? If you're struggling to see the positives in a situation, ask someone to help you collect the evidence. Or, if there really are few, if any, positives, think about what you can do to cope and not let your life spin out of control.

"I only get it right when I'm doing something so easy that anybody could do it."

These types of self-downing thoughts are examples of what's called *maximization/minimization.* You maximize the negative part of the situation, or you minimize the positive, or both. So, in a case like this, if you do something wrong you accept that you are a screw-up; the negative is confirmed and emphasized. If you get it right, you assume it's because you had some sort of advantage that others don't have; the positive is minimized. This keeps the negative belief intact.

When you're maximizing or minimizing, consider what you're *not* seeing. Ask yourself:

Can anybody really do the things I'm doing?

Have I completed difficult tasks in the past?

Am I overgeneralizing a small mistake to feel like a complete failure?

DESIGN A PERSONAL REALITY-CHECK EXPERIMENT

One way to increase your confidence in an alternative belief is to become a personal scientist in your own life. You can test your beliefs like scientists test hypotheses. Remember, your thoughts are just thoughts; they are hypotheses about yourself in the world.

There are several ways to create a behavioral experiment, depending on the thought. For thoughts about how others view you, or about your ideas compared to others, you can conduct a survey of people whose opinions you trust. You can ask, "Do you ever think that everyone else is more successful than you?" or "I tend to think that when I get it right, it must have been so easy that anyone can do it. Do you find that odd?"

For thoughts that confirm a particular interpretation of a situation to prove your belief about yourself, you can state an alternative hypothesis, such as, "Not everyone can do this thing that I'm good at." Then do a little sleuthing. Observe other people doing the same task and see what you learn; you might find they don't succeed as much as you.

For thoughts that people respond to you differently than they do to others, set a hypothesis. You might state, "Other people think I'm less capable than everyone else" or "Everyone treats me like I'm dumber than they are." Then do an observational study, looking objectively at how others react to different people. Listen in on conversations, when it is socially appropriate to do so, to gather data.

Do you observe people overexplaining to others? If so, consider whether it really means they think you are "dumb" when they do so to you. Do you observe that people don't say "thank you" when someone holds the door for them but just walk through? If so, consider that when people do the same to you, it may be that they aren't exceptionally polite—not that they don't respect you.

"Nothing I do will matter."

When you feel hopeless, this thought might keep running through your head. This is an example of fortune-telling. You predict the future with no evidence for it. Although you may have tried many things to feel better or make changes that haven't worked out, this doesn't mean it will always be so. Essentially, this is the difference between pessimism—expecting the worst—and optimism—expecting the best.

REALIZE NO ONE CAN PREDICT THE FUTURE

Being realistic means accepting that you don't know what will happen. A moment in the future could be good, bad, or neutral. Your past need not hold your thinking about the future hostage. Here's what you can do to reduce fortune-telling:

1. Remind yourself of times in the past when you've successfully influenced an outcome in your favor, and that you have not been 100 percent powerless to change situations.
2. Consider that life can surprise you; you don't know what will or will not happen. Not knowing can mean that something good or neutral can happen, not that only something bad can happen. Consider depressed fortune-telling like drunk texting—the message is likely to be garbled and regrettable. What you predict when you are in a depressed mode likely is not accurately reflecting every possibility.
3. Recognize that you may be downplaying the impact you have (maximizing or minimizing).

"If there is a downside, I will find it."

This thought is an example of selective abstraction, or seeing only one aspect of a situation instead of all the information available. Human beings are good at seeing what can make us unhappy or what threatens our safety. You may have become especially good at this throughout your life. Early trauma, losses, and the genetic makeup you came into the world with all influence this point of view. You may be thinking, "But it is bad! I'm not imagining it," and you would be right—in part.

TAKE IN THE BIGGER PICTURE

Usually there is either something good that you're not directing your attention to, or there are ways to cope with the bad that are hard for you to see. Rigid thinking may be at work, so evaluating your thoughts will be important. Here's what you can do:

1. Consider all of the possibilities in the bigger picture. Decide which possibilities may be true, including the worst ones. Consider how much you believe there is good as well as bad in the situation.

2. Look at what you might be able to do in the midst of the bad parts. For example, you can keep your eyes trained on the moment, you can focus on just getting through the moment, or you can reach out for help.

"I can't even . . . "

This overused phrase, applied to all sorts of situations, is an example of awfulizing or catastrophizing. It expresses an exasperation with people or situations that are most likely not as awful or terrible as the thought makes them seem. Ellis asserted that the way we talk to ourselves influences how we feel.

REDEFINE THE SITUATION

When you say things like "I can't" or "This is awful," you're giving yourself directions. These words can be more than mere expressions; they also reflect your frustration and exaggerate your feelings.

1. Instead of thinking something is awful, think of it as inconvenient or a bummer.
2. If you say, "I can't even . . . ," explore what you may be truly feeling. That might yield a thought like, "Well, I actually just find this really annoying [or angering or sad or whatever the feeling]."

"This should not be happening."

This type of thought is known as a should. Shoulds are demands we make on ourselves, others, or the world that usually don't fit with certain realities. Common should thoughts sound like, "It shouldn't be this hard," "I shouldn't be feeling this way," "You shouldn't act that way," or "That's not the way it should be—the world is so unfair." However, nothing dictates how things should be, only how they might be better or more desirable in a given situation.

IDENTIFY THE RULE . . . IF THERE IS ONE

When you're shoulding on the world, yourself, or others (as Ellis would say), the first step is to stop. Then, remind yourself that the situation could be fine, even better than expected. Nowhere is it written that anything should be one way or another. Life doesn't come with a rule book.

"If only I'd not done that, nothing bad would've happened."

This thinking is an example of hindsight bias. Have you ever gotten into a fender bender and then kicked yourself for taking the route in the first place? Hindsight bias. It means imagining that if you had done something differently, a better outcome would've resulted. The problem is, hindsight bias can leave you second-guessing your decisions.

What if you had moved to a different town? Found a different partner? Studied something else? Stayed in the job that didn't pay enough? With hindsight bias, we usually answer these what-if questions with something positive: Our life would have been better. But we don't really know this. In all of these situations, having made a different decision or taken a different action could have led to something much worse.

TEST WHAT-IF SCENARIOS

Ruminating about the past is common in depression. But hindsight bias results in regret, which leads to suffering. Learn to trust yourself and your past decisions.

1. Identify at least one unhelpful what-if belief that prevails in your thinking
2. Rather than finish the what-if with something better than your current situation, imagine two or three worst scenarios. For example, rather than having a fender bender, what if you'd taken a different route? Imagine that you could have run over a giant screw, blown out a tire, then spun out and hit a parked

car, totaling yours in the process. Is this any more realistic than the biased thought that it would have been better if you only did something different? No, but it allows you to examine many more possibilities than what you did was wrong.

3. Remember that you have today, and all the days following, to make new decisions. You can't redo bad decisions or decisions that had a bad result. Choose to live now rather than in the past. Do what you can to fix the bad outcome, and if you can't do anything because the outcome was permanent, offer yourself a little grace. You gain nothing by endlessly berating yourself; but you and those around you can gain a great deal when you commit to doing better from here forward.

DISCONNECT FROM YOUR THOUGHTS

Imagine your thoughts as "things," perhaps as little balloons. Observe their colors, sizes, whether they have longer or shorter strings. Since these thoughts are not facts, and they are not part of you, visually picture them outside of yourself . . . Picture those thoughts, those little balloons, drifting up into the air further and further from you once you let go of the string.

SAY "I'M HAVING THE THOUGHT THAT . . . "

Psychologist Steven Hayes and his ACT colleagues have a simple yet elegant way to easily practice defusion.[3] For one day, whenever you recognize a troubling thought, say to yourself, "I'm having the thought that . . . " For example, if you think, "I was so horrible to my sister back then," change it to "I'm having the thought that I was horrible to my sister back then."

In the first instance, the thought sounds like a fact and makes that experience from your past a present reality. Humans are capable of feeling today what we felt decades ago by "reliving" it through the monologues in our heads. In the second instance, the current reality is just that a thought has come into your mind; the here and now is not consumed by reliving, but just experiencing a thought. Some of the bite is taken away.

CONSIDER ALTERNATIVES

You probably don't recognize how much your unhelpful thinking keeps your focus narrow. It might seem obvious that there are alternative ways of looking at things, but when you're depressed, your scope shrinks. Think of your mood as creating a glaucoma of the mind; what you see gets smaller and smaller until it's hard to see more than one option.

Thankfully, you can exercise your brain to see things more broadly. At first, it may seem like you're forcing yourself to consider alternatives that you don't really believe, and that's okay. As one example, when you recognize that the monologue in your head is particularly negative, say to yourself, "This is only one moment. I may feel differently shortly." Notice that I'm not suggesting that you tell yourself that rainbows will come out tomorrow and that all is well with your soul. Just let yourself believe different self-talk. It's a possible alternative, after all.

Consider as many alternatives as you can. Over time, you might find evidence that supports alternative thoughts. You may come to realize that you've been seeing things in a rigid way, which is not the only possible way of viewing the world.

GOT MILK? ANOTHER WAY TO DEFUSE FROM YOUR THOUGHTS

Another exercise that offers you an alternative way to think about your thoughts and defuse from them at the same time is to do a bit of wordplay. In ACT, the exercise is to take a word like "milk" and think about what it conjures in your mind. Spoken once, the word brings up thoughts of a cold, silky, white beverage. As a child who grew up on a dairy farm, it brings up images of home, my mother straining out cream, and feelings of comfort.

Now say "milk" repeatedly—and quickly—over and over again. The word becomes something like "mluk, mkk, mlll, lkk"—gibberish, nonsense. This is one way to disentangle yourself from the emotions the thought brings. The thoughts that you have fused with are words in your head. When they make you suffer, it's helpful to remove the power they hold by defusing from them.

STOP THE EARWORM

Sometimes thoughts just keep swirling through your head. You may be rehashing an experience that made you feel hurt in some way. This particular thought is like having a song stuck in your head, an earworm. Trying to stop the earworm by ignoring it is rarely successful.

A surefire way to stop an annoying earworm is to start singing a different song. Listen to something else. Refocus your attention. This is also helpful if you're stuck in repetitive negative thoughts about yourself, other people, or the world, when there is really nothing you can do to change who you are, they are, or how the world is at that moment.

If singing isn't helpful, attend to something that can be. Shift your attention by focusing deliberately—or "mindfully"—on the current moment or task. Notice the sights, smells, textures, and sounds all around you; intentionally focus on them. Don't worry about whether you have lost the earworm, because if you stop to think about whether you've been successful at moving on from it, you're likely to bring it back.

BECOME NONJUDGMENTAL

Start looking at yourself and your thoughts with a little more compassion and a little less judgment. Judging yourself for being given a lackluster life, or for being given everything that you never had to work for, will lead to the same outcome: judgment that is usually too harsh and unfair. So start by letting go of those judgments. As with the previous strategy, you can see them as balloons that you let drift away into the sky. You can also let go of self-critical thoughts by creating some distance from them, as described next.

Living Well

- You can develop a new, healthier relationship with your thoughts.
- You can decenter and objectively evaluate your thoughts, which gets

you in the practice of thinking more broadly and frees you from rigidity, which can be difficult for your mental well-being.

- You can make decisions with more ease and confidence. You can stop the shoulds that keep you grasping at the way something must be done, or you can remember that hindsight is also prone to bias.
- You can practice defusing from your thoughts by repeating words over and over until they are gibberish, or by telling yourself that "I'm having the thought that . . . "

PART TWO

navigating daily life with depression

4

keeping up with self-care

It's easy and common to ignore yourself when you're feeling depressed. Sometimes all you can do is the least you can do. Doing even the basics can seem difficult, but it's important to care for yourself. It's worth repeating that, as in an airplane, it's wise to put on your oxygen mask before assisting others.

The message you're sending to yourself if you're staying in bed, not bathing, wearing dirty clothing, or staying in pajamas all day is that you are not worth the bother or that life is not worth the bother. That is a negative message to convey, and engaging in this mood-dependent behavior will only make you feel worse and worse.

You may feel shut down, not care, or have thoughts that you don't deserve basic necessities. Allowing yourself to avoid activity keeps the emptiness and painful thoughts under your skin. But caring for yourself sends a different message: that you are someone who is important.

What Does Minimal Self-Care Look Like?

If you're meeting your goal of getting out of bed, but you're not taking care of yourself or basic household tasks, you can set a new goal of maintaining minimal self-care. Acting from the outside in—doing basic self-care, like putting your feet on the floor—will accomplish several things.

You've probably had the experience of feeling pretty awful when ill with a flu or fever. And you can probably recall feeling physically better when you showered and put on clean clothing. Even if those clean clothes were pajamas. We will use this approach—doing a few basic things to help us feel better—when getting out of bed may be the only win of the day.

Doing basic self-care is important for so many reasons. It helps get you activated and engaged in your life. It also reinforces the idea that you are worth being taken care of. Your depressed brain may tell you otherwise, but as with any urge toward mood-dependent behavior, you can act from the outside—doing these simple self-care activities to shift, even a little, how you feel or think on the inside.

So what's the minimum you can do for yourself? Here's a list of basic self-care behaviors that you could choose from, or choose all of them:

Personal Hygiene

- Get out of bed and go to the toilet when you first feel a need, rather than waiting until you have no choice
- Wash your face with a washcloth and soap, or simply splash water on your face and towel dry
- Rinse your mouth with a mouth rinse or mouthwash
- Brush your teeth
- Run a comb or brush through your hair
- If you shave your face regularly, shave
- Give yourself a sponge bath
- Wash your hair
- Take a shower
- Trim your fingernails and toenails
- Put on clean underwear

- Dress in clean "everyday" clothes
- Put on some makeup
- Paint your nails
- Take a bubble bath
- Use lotion on your skin
- Do a few calisthenics
- Stretch
- Do yoga
- Take a walk
- Open and close your hands to relax your fingers
- Get a haircut
- Get a manicure
- Use a face cleansing mask
- Massage your own shoulders or neck

Sustenance

- Drink a glass of water
- Make a cup of tea or coffee
- Drink a glass of juice
- Toast one or two slices of bread and eat it
- Eat a bowl of cold cereal
- Eat a health bar
- Boil or fry an egg or two
- Make instant oatmeal
- Cook hot cereal
- Leave your house to get take-out
- Sit in a coffee shop to eat
- Go to a restaurant for a full breakfast
- Go to the grocery store
- Buy your favorite food

Interpersonal Connection (If You Do Not Live Alone)

- Say good morning to the other people in your house
- Sit with someone and watch a morning TV show
- Sit with someone and read your phone
- Offer to make your housemate a cup of tea or coffee
- If you have children, put out breakfast cereal and milk for them
- Sit with your children—or other housemates and eat a small breakfast
- Fix lunch for your children
- Walk your children to the bus stop or to school
- Offer to drive someone to work

Interpersonal Connection (If You Live Alone)

- Call a friend
- Send a text to a loved one
- If you have a pet, give them a snuggle
- Write a note to someone, even if you don't plan to send it
- Look at your social media page*
- Post a comment on a social media page*

Add anything else that is relevant to you.

Should you decide to post something, think carefully about letting others know that you're struggling; generally, it's not recommended. You might get empathic responses, but you also might feel too exposed in the long run, which can lead to wanting to avoid friends—and this is the opposite of a self-care goal.

*The suggestions regarding social media come with a caveat. When you see what others are posting on social media it may be a catalyst for you to make comparisons and spiral into ruminations over your own distress and others' great lives. Remember that people usually post photos of their peak moments, not of cleaning the bathroom. These moments aren't a part of their everyday life.

How Do I Make Self-Care Stick?

The best way to make your self-care tasks a habit is to do them regularly. Over time, the habit will stick. I've found that the very best way to get started with a habit is to plan for it. In this case, I recommend filling out a Self-Care Plan (see the next page) in advance to schedule things that will give you a sense of accomplishment or pleasure. You may use the one provided (extra charts may be downloaded from *www.guilford.com/martell3-materials*). Jot down the self-care task you will do and at what time. Then check off when the task is completed.

There are several ways to approach your plan. One way is to schedule just one or two activities that you repeat over the course of a week. If you completed the Activity–Mood Chart (Chapter 3), you can pick a self-care activity that made you feel a little better. You can schedule the activities at various times or plan the same activity at the same time on several different days of the week.

Doing Self-Care Even When You Don't Feel Like It

In Chapter 2, we introduced the concept of acting as if; return there for a refresher. You'll be relying on this strategy for most of the tips that follow. Initially you will feel as if you're putting on an act, because, in fact, you are—and that is how you start. With basic self-care, there is nothing wrong with going through the motions as long as doing so increases the likelihood that you ultimately feel better.

The metaphor of learning to play an instrument is apropos to this idea. Consider learning the guitar. There are several "finger stretch" exercises that involve playing scales up and down the neck of the guitar or using different finger positions to play notes on all of the strings. It sounds nothing like music. It doesn't feel like playing the guitar. It's difficult at first. However, over time, the student of the guitar builds flexibility, and motor memory for the various fingering and frets. Eventually the student can master the instrument and play or compose music.

SELF-CARE PLAN

Time	Self-Care Task	Completed? (Yes or No)
12 A.M.		
1 A.M.		
2 A.M.		
3 A.M.		
4 A.M.		
5 A.M.		
6 A.M.		
7 A.M.		
8 A.M.		
9 A.M.		
10 A.M.		
11 A.M.		
12 P.M.		
1 P.M.		
2 P.M.		
3 P.M.		
4 P.M.		
5 P.M.		
6 P.M.		
7 P.M.		
8 P.M.		
9 P.M.		
10 P.M.		
11 P.M.		

Whatever it is that you're doing to go through the motions is likely to work like the guitar exercise. It's not going to be the loveliest music of your life; it might just be a boring exercise. But you're building behavioral flexibility, and acting as if you can cope with the various needs of your life. Over time the flexibility will allow you to truly cope and to feel better as you break patterns of avoiding hard tasks, retreating from negative emotions, and hating on yourself. With acting as if, you'll soon find that little engagements keep you moving forward. Each small step you take toward minimal self-care adds good habits to your routine.

"I don't have the energy to exercise."

Both depression and physical illness reduce activity. It's important to rest when our bodies need it. And it's equally important to move when our bodies are well. The ABCs presented in Chapter 2 can help you assess whether you really need the rest because you're unwell, or whether you're feeling lethargic because you're in a depressive mood. This can be hard to determine. You can also see how you feel after a little exercise. It need not be a walk around your block, although it can be that. You might just take a few steps outside your front door.

MOVE TO STAY MOTIVATED

We aren't always motivated to do our best, and sometimes we aren't motivated to do anything. You might say, "My body feels heavy and weak all the time, so how am I supposed to go for a walk?" But as I've mentioned before, we don't need to wait until we feel up to doing things to do them, because motivation follows action. Experts in *motivational interviewing,* a therapeutic process for helping people change bad habits, help people move from contemplating change to taking action. They don't give anyone a feel-good moment to get them to act, they simply help them to make decisions to change. Once you take the first steps to change, the rest of the steps can follow.

Exercise of any sort is a great place to start. We know that physical activity alone can improve mood. You won't walk yourself out of depression, but you can certainly begin to take some steps that will give you small successes. Small successes lead to further successes.

- Fill out a Self-Care Plan chart and schedule when you will do some form of physical movement or exercise.
- Establish a short daily routine to move your body.
- Check in with yourself and do what your body allows you to do (you may wish to consult your health care provider if you plan to start any type of new, strenuous activity).
- Give yourself some type of reward each time you complete the activity. For example, allow yourself to eat a sweet snack afterward. Write a congratulatory note to yourself on a postcard and post it on your refrigerator. Call someone with whom you enjoy talking. Go out for a nice meal. Or include the reward *during* the activity by inviting someone to join you in the task.

"If I don't walk a mile or at least exercise 30 minutes a day, it isn't worth doing at all."

Don't fall into the trap of *thinking* you need to do an entire activity before actually *doing* any of it. This type of thinking—called *all-or-nothing thinking*—keeps people stuck in all-or-nothing action.

AVOID ALL-OR-NOTHING ACTION

Most writing coaches will tell their students who are having difficulty writing to write just one paragraph. If you want to exercise but aren't able to do a full workout, for whatever reason, it's still useful to do what you can.

This dilemma can occur for many activities, not just exercise. Another example might be, "If I don't get my hair cut, why bother washing and combing it?" Or "If I don't have all the ingredients to make my favorite dinner, I shouldn't make anything." That is all-or-nothing thinking and behaving.

You can make your life a little nicer by doing these things—even a small part of it. Combing your hair is a nonverbal way of treating yourself like you're prepared to meet the world, even if you don't really think that you are. You can still eat well even if it's not the meal you were craving.

"My body's not what it used to be, so why bother taking care of it?"

A common trap is to have expectations of yourself that are outdated. The physical prowess one has at age 22 is different from the physical prowess one has at 50, and expecting to still act, perform, and look like 22 when one is 50 is a losing proposition. Similarly, when you're depressed, you might think, "I used to be able to do so much more, before I felt this way," or "I used to be so much better looking." These are also traps.

STAY IN THE PRESENT MOMENT

When you start to compare your now self with your then self, it's time to practice getting out of your head. Stop and recognize that you have pulled away from the moment. You've distanced yourself from the physical activity that could bring some minimal pleasure and enjoyment, and instead you're attending to the mental activity in your head. Accept that this is what your mind has done, and bring your attention back to whatever task you were engaging in.

You may tell yourself that you are your only standard, that you don't need to live up to anyone else's expectations. But you might underestimate the way you've internalized certain standards put in place by marketing from the entertainment and beauty industries. Unwittingly, your own standard may have become an impossible expectation that is just not you—and never will be. Live according to what you value, rather than living up to arbitrary high standards.

"I don't feel like calling the dentist."

Fear or anxiety around the dentist is common. Many people don't like going even for the simplest of procedures, like getting teeth cleaned. They may not even feel like calling the dentist to set up an appointment that is months in the future. But when you're depressed, putting off such a task may be due to a lack of energy as much as actual fear of the visit itself. Put another way, when you're having difficulty keeping up with self-care of the basic, daily variety, adding in something that requires professional service can feel like a whole other mountain to conquer.

This is exactly when you need to act according to a plan, not a feeling or mood.

ACT ACCORDING TO PLAN

You can manage this. Putting together all of the strategies presented so far can help you when you really don't feel like doing something. Make the calendar your friend. You don't have to schedule the appointment now, but rather use the calendar or a phone reminder to schedule the first step: looking up the phone number for your dentist. When you reach that date on the calendar, find the number, no matter how you feel. Once you've done that you have a success! You've acted on a plan not a feeling.

Then, you can plan the next step. Now that you have the phone number, you can schedule a date on the calendar to call. Or you can set a time to store the number of the dentist in your phone, and call later. You might be thinking, "This is silly, I should just call!" But that's your pre-depression standards talking. If "just calling" was so simple, you would have done it.

Acting according to a plan takes intention and commitment. And since motivation follows action, the activity may need to be very easy, require a brief amount of time, and give you a result that gets you one step closer to your goal.

"There's no way I'm going to shower today."

At one point or another, we all feel as if we can't bear something, as if there's just no way it'll happen. But the body can surprise us. And, as you're learning in this book, getting through depression is less about your mood and more about action.

GO ONE STEP FURTHER

Try this experiment: Whatever you feel capable of right now, do it, then go one step further. For example, if you wake up and you honestly feel that washing your face is the best you can do, go ahead and do it—then see if you can add moisturizer. Or put on some lipstick or trim your beard. Try some additional small thing and notice how rewarding it feels to know you can take on a new challenge, no matter how tiny.

"I'm sleeping too much" or "I'm not sleeping enough."

Sleep is often disrupted when someone is depressed, and disrupted sleep can be a catalyst for depression. Sleep is important. There are treatments for people who suffer from primary insomnia, and seeking professional help may be an important step if this applies to you. Some strategies can work for you whether you're having difficulty falling or staying asleep, or whether you're sleeping too much. Not all strategies will be effective for both. When you're depressed and not sleeping or sleeping too much (hypersomnia), you can use strategies to act from the outside in to your advantage in getting back to a good sleep routine. But when you're sleeping too little, we recommend not going to bed until you feel sleepy. In this situation, relying on your feeling at bedtime is important.

USE EXTERNAL MONITORS

Timers and alarm clocks can be helpful to help you wake up in the morning. They can also be helpful for getting to bed at a regular time, especially if you sleep too little or too much. Don't go to bed until the timer goes off. Ultimately, the goal here is to get yourself into a routine so that eventually you won't need the timer; your body will tell you when it's time to go to bed.

AVOID NAPPING

A good long nap can feel restorative after a long week. Under usual conditions, this is a lovely way to treat yourself. However, if you're dealing with insomnia, napping will interfere with your ability to be sleepy at bedtime. If you're sleeping too much, a nap will just contribute to lethargy. Here are a few tips to beat the pull to nap:

- Don't sit in your bed or in a particularly comfortable chair or sofa.
- Find an activity that will hold your interest.
- Avoid passive activities like watching television or scrolling on your phone.
- Splash cold water on your face.
- If you're physically able, take a short walk outdoors.
- Get out of your house completely.
- Go to a café, but avoid having caffeine late in the day, as it also can disrupt your sleep schedule.
- Go to a store to just browse.
- Call a friend or relative.
- Walk around the room when you're on the phone rather than sitting.
- Play with your pet or your child.

Like an itch that will eventually go away even if you can't scratch it, the pull to nap will eventually go away if you redirect your attention. You might need to go to bed a little earlier than you might have before you were dealing with hypersomnia, but the point here is to sleep on a schedule.

EASE UP ON *SHOULD* LANGUAGE

Recommended sleep amounts are easy to find online. You may even own a smart watch that will congratulate you when you've reached your sleep goals. That's all well and good, but it can also send you careening down the hill of the *shoulds.* As the late psychologist Albert Ellis used to say, "Where is it written?"[1] Sure, recommended sleep amounts are provided by experts. But those figures are based on optimal conditions. Your condition, at present, isn't optimal. You may be struggling, and therefore reaching a certain standard isn't possible. Sure, you can work toward your ideal goal, but recognize that healthy aspirations keep us moving forward; they aren't hard and fast rules that we are obligated to follow even when circumstances change. Allowing yourself flexibility and grace will help you feel better—and probably sleep better—in the long run.

"I'm eating too much" or "I'm not eating enough."

Food is complicated. Many people in the world don't have access to enough food, while for others there is an abundance of food. Meals may be eaten together with family and friends, or they may be ritualized in various religious traditions. Food can be used to reward good behavior or can be taken away to punish bad behavior. We judge one another and ourselves about food, the amount of food we eat, or the types of foods we eat. When we experience strong emotions, our desire for food is impacted.

All of this happens with or without depression. With depression, changes in eating patterns and appetite are common. Here are strategies to help if you're struggling with appetite. However, if you're experiencing serious difficulties with eating and appetite, or believe you may have an eating disorder, it's recommended that you seek professional support.

EAT THROUGHOUT THE DAY

It can be challenging to eat with some regularity when you're busy or when you're depressed. The downward cycle of depression—being less active, staying in bed, avoiding simple tasks—can also result in not having food in your home, not preparing meals, or not feeling like eating. Or you might have a cupboard full of convenient foods that don't really satisfy you. Having three balanced meals a day gives you proper nourishment to perform better—though we know it can be particularly challenging when you have no appetite.

When it comes to food, acting from the outside in—which is literally what you must do—is a strategy to keep up with reasonable nutritional needs. Plan to eat on a schedule. It might be difficult to eat a full meal when your appetite is suppressed, but eating at set times rather than waiting to be hungry will help you stay nourished. Even if you're not hungry, eat something small, like a piece of fruit or a protein shake.

If you're overeating, you can still take advantage of a schedule to eat throughout the day. Choose smaller portions of nutritious meals and allow a light snack between meals only when the timer rings. You may crave more, you may feel unsatisfied, but keep acting from the outside in and, over time, the craving will go away as you develop a different habit.

LOOK AT THE FUNCTION OF YOUR EATING HABITS

How is eating serving you? Understanding the ABCs of eating is as helpful as understanding the function of any behavior. Is undereating or overeating a way of numbing your emotions? Is zoning out the consequence (C) for you? Under what circumstances are you most likely to turn to food? Do you turn to food to make you feel loved when you're lonely? On the other hand, do you avoid eating because it makes you feel noble? Or because you think that not eating is a healthy choice when it isn't?

FIND AN ALTERNATIVE TO STRESS EATING

If you've recognized that you eat to manage stress, try doing other things so that you don't fall into the same repeating pattern of feeling stressed, eating or overeating, feeling guilty or physically sick, then feeling more stressed. Neuroscientist Kelly Lambert suggests that the modern world allows, perhaps demands, us to be less active and may result in more instances of depression. Rewards that require physical activity can help. Lambert, in her book *Lifting Depression,* refers to research indicating that activities like knitting have been shown to reduce anxiety. Can you try an activity that uses your hands and produces a product, to help manage your depression and stress?

"Why bother to look good?"

When you feel depressed it may be difficult to see the point in anything, particularly in taking time to make yourself up or dress nicely. But the principle of working from the outside in applies here as well. You don't need to feel like you're worth getting your hair styled or a pedicure or putting on a nice outfit before leaving the house; you need to act as if you are. Treating yourself as worth something can make you feel worth something.

DITCH THE NEGATIVE STORY

Guilt, shame, self-blame—all can seem like apparent justifications for treating yourself badly or giving up on yourself. Negative beliefs about yourself confirm to you that you don't deserve to look good, to be admired, to give a care. However, what you've done in the past is done. You can decide to start making amends, if needed, and improve your life by taking simple steps of self-care.

You also may be engaging in some of the unhelpful cognitive distortions we addressed in Chapter 3. Notice whether you are overfocusing on the negative and ignoring the positive about yourself, or holding onto *shoulds* and absolute demands of yourself. If so, change the story and change the way you treat yourself, even a little.

CREATE THE SIMPLEST PLEASURE

Noticing moments that are pleasurable can have big impacts on your mental health. Sure, that nail polish isn't going to fix anything, but it can give you a little boost when you look at your pretty hands. When very little gives you pleasure—what we called anhedonia—take time to really notice things that are enjoyable, or even merely neutral, like the way the color of your shirt complements your complexion, or the taste of each lick of an ice cream cone on a hot day. Dwell in the experience of something that could or that once did give you pleasure. You don't need to fake the enjoyment, just engage in the moment.

Billy's Story

Billy felt as though he had been depressed most of his life. He could remember thinking about future troubles when he was just a young boy. While he never was diagnosed as a child, when he sought an online therapist at age 32, he thought back on his life and found it lacking in joy. He had been married for seven years, but then had a brief extramarital affair which ruined his marriage. The relationship he'd started during the marriage didn't last either.

After his divorce, Billy moved into a small studio apartment in a rundown part of the city where he lived. The apartment building was tucked between two larger buildings, and the only window in the main part of the apartment faced a wall. The tiny kitchenette's small window looked over power lines and a parking lot. He thought this studio was like a prison cell and believed this was what he deserved.

Four months after his divorce, he was so miserable that he frequently was late for his job as an automobile detailer. He also was very slow at work, and his boss needed to assign someone to assist him in order to get the jobs done. After missing four days of work in a row and only calling in two out of the four times, his boss, who considered Billy a friend, told him that he must either get help or be fired. Billy couldn't imagine going to see anyone for help, but he contacted a therapist anyway.

During Billy's first session, the therapist provided Billy with a diagnosis of depression and encouraged Billy to ask his boss for a brief leave of absence. The boss agreed to hold Billy's job but could not pay him during his leave. Billy thought he could manage on his savings for about three weeks.

Being on leave allowed Billy to give in to the inertia that had overwhelmed him. Apart from using the bathroom or getting up to eat potato chips or crackers when he felt a little hunger, Billy just stayed in bed. His beard grew scruffy and his hair became greasy. When he glanced in the mirror early one morning he saw someone who looked more like he belonged on a park bench than in the smallest studio apartment. Billy's therapist also noticed the deterioration during their session, which Billy joined via his laptop while staying in bed. The therapist asked Billy if he was willing to get out of bed and take a shower. Reluctantly, Billy agreed.

When he finished his therapy session, Billy ran a hot shower and laid out clean underwear, jeans and a T-shirt. The shower felt good. It was like having a good wash after working outdoors on a hot, sweaty day. Water running over his hair and the back of his neck felt relaxing. More relaxing than staying in bed. Once he had cleaned up and dressed, he made a cup of instant coffee. This was the first coffee he'd had in several days and drinking it eased the headache he'd been nursing. He found cereal in his cabinet, and the milk in his refrigerator—still within its use-by date and not sour—was good, so he poured himself a bowl.

Billy thought he might return to his bed, but when he smelled his dirty linens, the contrast with the clean feeling he had post shower was stark. He decided to sit at the small table in the kitchenette and play a game on his phone. He didn't feel up to taking his linens to the laundry, but he did manage to change his sheets and pillowcase before going back to bed in the afternoon. He wasn't miraculously better, but he did feel less gross and ill. This was an important first step in taking care of himself and then working with his therapist to manage the guilt and shame he was feeling about his divorce.

Living Well

- Self-care is not only important for maintaining your physical health; it's also important for your mental health. When you ignore basic care, you're treating yourself like someone who deserves to be ignored.
- Take small steps to get back into good healthy habits with sleep, food, and exercise. Doing so builds momentum. Remember, motivation follows action.

5

handling daily chores

Few of us look forward to chores. So it's no wonder that depression has made these tasks last on your list. When you already don't enjoy things that are "supposed" to be enjoyable, it can be particularly difficult to have to take up the drudgery of daily chores. It can feel unbearable.

Fortunately, there's no rule that says you have to like doing something to do it. In fact, it's how the vast majority of us are able to maintain a habitable environment. If you've ever had a pet, for example, you're familiar with the feeling of not wanting to clean up their messes in or around your house—but you do it anyway. In this chapter, we'll look at some strategies for dealing with chores that aren't enjoyable but necessary.

How Do I Chip Away at What Needs to Get Done?

There are many ways chores can keep you grounded and engaged rather than annoyed by the hassle. We'll draw on many of the strategies offered in Chapters 1, 2, and 3—because they work. If some start to sound repetitive, well, it's because they are; research tells us that frequent reminders help with task completion. In this chapter, you'll see how to apply those strategies directly to issues in your living space.

Here are a few things to keep in mind before we talk about specific activities:

What to Do versus What to Get Done

I'm a big supporter of the saying, "Some things you do, and some things you get done." There's flexibility built into this saying. Some tasks you may really get into, and others you have to get out of the way.

Begin to notice that the same activities can mean different things for you on different days or even at different times of the day. For example, on one evening after a long day at work you might find washing dishes relaxing. You can let the warmth of the water on your hands bring you into the present moment and not worry about anything else. That is what we would call *something you do.*

On a different evening, you may come home from work, fix something to eat, see the dirty dishes, and decide all you need cleaned is your coffee pot and a mug so you can have a freshly brewed beverage in the morning. So you wash only those two items. This is *something you get done.*

Usually, the tasks that we *get done* take less time; when we're in a hurry, we get them out of the way. Things that *we do* typically take more care and time; we're likely invested in the process, even if we wouldn't call it particularly enjoyable.

Working on a Task versus Finishing a Task

Working on a task is as important as actually finishing a task. People tend to be results oriented, especially in parts of the Western world and most particularly in North America. In Chapter 4 we emphasized setting goals for developing healthy habits (process oriented) rather than setting goals about losing weight or gaining muscle (outcome oriented). The same principle applies here. When there are chores hanging over your head, just working on the task is the start you need.

Let's say your home is a mess. It's daunting and you have no motivation to do anything. It's not realistic to tell yourself you're going to *finish* cleaning up the mess. But it's realistic to tell yourself that you can *work* on it. So look at what you can work on: picking up dirty clothing that has been dropped in various places throughout the house. You might also get some dusting out of the way after you've picked up the clothes and maybe put away some other clutter. Is your house clean? Well, no. Is it better than before? Yes. Did you *work on* the task despite not being able to *finish* it and in spite of your lack of motivation? Yes. You might notice that this is a perfect example of acting from the outside in, discussed in previous chapters.

It's worth pointing out that *working on* a task means being okay with taking smaller steps or tackling only parts of an activity, as part of the *process*. You may, therefore, need to deal with possible self-judgments, *should* thinking, and the pressured guilt of not having "success" until you've completed everything (the *outcome*). We address these experiences in this chapter.

Another bonus when you focus on the process rather than the outcome is that you will also be more likely to stay in the present moment. This can allow you to focus your attention on the experience, such as noticing (and maybe even enjoying) the comforting smell of detergent when doing laundry or the crisper view through the window after you've wiped the glass. Do the task mindfully. It will help to keep your shadowy thoughts at bay and keep you more focused on living from now to now.

Doing Household Chores Even When You Don't Feel Like It

A scene from the M. Knight Shyamalan movie *The Village* is apt here. Two teenage girls, wearing pioneer dresses, are sweeping a dusty porch on a log cabin. Their brooms look to be made from straw. It appears to be a boring, miserable, repetitive chore. They look at one another momentarily and each one takes turns twirling in a circle and they laugh. That little image is great, because sometimes you just need to do a little dance while you're doing something you find to be drudgery.

Audio technology allows us to listen to something pleasant while working, to make the task more enjoyable. You can play your favorite music as loud as your environment allows. You can use earbuds to call someone you enjoy talking to and chat as you work. You can listen to an engaging podcast or mystery audiobook.

If having company makes tasks easier for you, perhaps agree to do the chore together. Whatever can lighten your experience of the task, seek it out. The suggestions for the common situations below can help.

"How is my house not going to be messy if I can't bear to clean?"

If you're not someone who enjoys cleaning, and you don't find it to be calming, trying to organize a messy house can feel like a classic Sisyphean task, as meaningless as rolling a boulder up a hill only to have it roll back down. It can feel as if it takes a great deal of effort to clean, and very little effort to get it messy. If you're in a fortunate position to afford a housekeeping service, problem solved. You only have to take action to call in the cleaner. When you don't have that option, here are some things to consider.

LEAVE A LITTLE MESS

Maybe you can leave some small messes around. For instance, dust bunnies—those little tumbleweeds of dust and hair with the cute name that are not cute at all. Do you get annoyed seeing the dust bunnies, or cobwebs, or a pile of papers on your dining room table? Perhaps you can learn to live with them. Because sometimes feeling overwhelmed by cleaning is approaching the problem from the wrong side.

These things reflect a home that's simply dusty or cluttered—but not unsanitary. Try letting your house be a little untidy. Go ahead and sit on the sofa and read, even though the dusty coffee table is in front of you. Remind yourself that you can live with an imperfect house. Eventually, you'll schedule time to take steps to tidy up.

LET GO OF *SHOULD* THINKING

Once again, the *shoulds* need to go! We cause ourselves so much misery and guilt with our *should* beliefs. Sure, it's a good thing to abide by rules such as you should not kill people and you should pay the bills in order to keep your lights on. However, there is no stone tablet saying "Thou shalt not do something that you enjoy unless thou hast a tidy house." The founder of Methodism, John Wesley, may have said in his sermon "cleanliness is next to godliness," but that is a very tall order. Sure, life might be more convenient when certain things are clean, but the demand is what's problematic. It's unreasonable to live by a rule that you must always have a spotless home. Let it go.

PICK ONE THING YOU CAN TOLERATE

Keep up the practice of acting according to a goal rather than a mood. When your mood and the heaviness of depression loom and you want to stay in bed, you can still decide on one thing that you can tolerate doing. Even if you think you've reached capacity, you can still do one small thing. See the task not as mopping, for example, but as acting toward the goal of having a clean floor. These are a few ideas of small things you can do regardless of your mood:

- Clean one object. Perhaps dust off a picture frame.
- Put away a tool that has been sitting on your counter.
- Wipe the soap spots off your bathroom faucet.
- Sweep a cobweb out of one corner.
- Water a plant.
- Fold a few pieces of laundry.
- Vacuum one room.

DO ONE THING REGULARLY

It's worth coming back to this suggestion when it comes to keeping up at home. Picking one task and developing a habit of doing it with regularity will make the task less daunting. The saying "Never go to bed with a dirty sink" comes to mind. What's one thing you can get behind? Maybe it's charging your devices every night or wiping the bathroom sink every morning. When you do something by habit, you don't need to think about it, you just get up and do it.

Setting chores in a schedule can also help. Pay bills on a certain day of the month, do laundry on a specific day of the week, and so forth.

Doing it regularly builds the habit. At some point, it may even feel awkward *not* to do it; you'll feel as if there is something left undone—and you'd be right. That said, neglecting the chore occasionally is okay! These ideas are about helping you keep moving forward and living well, not giving you tasks that you obediently do without fail.

"I let the snail mail and email pile up . . . but who doesn't?"

If depression leaves you distracted and inattentive, if lethargy causes you to toss mail in a pile on a table, or if you have hundreds of unread emails, you might not care enough to bother with any of it. Sometimes it can be good to give yourself a break. As we stated earlier, sometimes it's okay to let the dust bunnies settle. On the other hand, some things that go unattended could have consequences that will make your life harder in the long run.

SORT IMMEDIATELY

Keep the recycling bin near your front door. Sort the junk from the necessities as soon as you bring your mail into your home. The junk you can get rid of right away. Try having two receptacles for the mail you bring in: one for the clearly necessary mail—a bill, an important notice, or personal correspondence—and one for the mail that doesn't seem urgent but that you'll need to open eventually. Start here, then look at the dates they were mailed and open older mail to catch up with time-limited items.

USE A FILTER

With email, you can go into the app's settings or preferences and set up email filters. A filter can divert email into specific folders of your choosing. For instance, all correspondence from a child's school can go into a "School" folder you set up, mail from utility companies can go into a "Bills" folder, and so on. You also don't have to do this alone. In the next chapter, we'll discuss how others can be a support; most of us know someone who's a techie and willing to help. Doing this initial round of vetting can change how you see what might look like a daunting task (a pile of unopened envelopes or a long list of unread emails), and the task will seem more manageable.

SELECT ONE DAY A MONTH

Pick a number from 1 to 28. Got it? That's the day every month you must open your mail or unsubscribe from one or more junk email senders. Keep a recycling bin nearby to get rid of all the other junk mail and toss it, or put the envelopes through a shredder if you prefer.

"I can't keep up with anything—how can I pay my bills on time?"

You may not have a problem with mail piling up, but it may be hard for you to sit down and take care of necessary things like paying bills. The issue may be that you need to make hard decisions about what you can afford and which bills need to take priority. If money is tight or if handling finances is challenging, you may understandably have a strong urge to avoid the entire process. It might be helpful to call creditors and explain if you're having difficulty affording multiple payments.

AUTOMATE PAYMENTS

If you know you'll be able to afford monthly bills, technology can be your best friend. Set up an automatic bill-pay program with your bank. If you're intimidated by technology, have a friend or family member help you set this up if you don't know how. You can also go into a financial institution and have an employee help you set this up.

"There are too many chores to do—what's wrong with just watching television?"

By now, you're aware that avoidance is understandable, especially when you're depressed. Perhaps that's one reason escapist television so often features people with magic powers. Blink your eyes, twitch your nose, say a magic word, or wave your hand, and your home is sparkling clean. If only life were that easy. Imagination is the only place any of us can snap our fingers and make all things right. When you find yourself zoning out because there is so much to be done, gently remind yourself that consistent avoidance causes more harm eventually. See if you can do one thing, like take out the trash, before sitting in front of a screen. Then see if you can do one more thing, like put a fresh trash bag in the can.

PAY ATTENTION TO ONE ACTIVITY

Do one chore at a time and don't worry about the rest. Really engage in the task at hand. For example, vacuuming the floor doesn't seem like a task you'd want to pay attention to. Try paying attention to the pattern on the rug you're vacuuming or the grain in a wood floor. If you have a solid-color carpet, notice how the vacuum cleaner makes trails as you move along. This exercise can work even if you have an automated vacuum; just spend time watching the little helper move around your home and get the task done.

"I hate this place . . . why bother to fix it up?"

You may not live in your dream home. You may live in a place that is far less than you would choose, but you might not have a choice. It may be a rental that you don't plan to invest money in. But you can set up a space just for you. It might be one half of one room with a favorite chair, a small table, and a sunny window that makes you feel at ease. Make it yours.

CALL ON YOUR VALUES

Rather than giving up on where you live or focusing on what you don't like, make time to do things in your home that are consistent with your values. If maintaining friendships is consistent with your values but you aren't comfortable inviting people to your home, plan times to call friends so that you stay in touch. You don't need to love your home to do what's important to you. If you're a parent and value time with your children, set up an area for games or plan popcorn and movie nights.

You can also try simple things that could make being in your home more pleasant. For example, if your nice things are put away because you have young children, try making your place more appealing in another way, perhaps with diffusers, incense, or candles, if you live somewhere that is safe to have those things. If you don't want to burn things in your home, find a cleaning product with a fragrance you like or an essential oil. You might put several of these strategies to work and mindfully bake a batch of chocolate chip cookies to give your place a homey feeling—even if you use the prepared kind of dough.

ADD VISUAL APPEAL

Get a small plant that you can watch grow. If you can afford to buy little things that speak to you, make the place yours. If you have the means to actually do a bit more, choose an entire room and make it one you can enjoy. A new coat of paint and a piece or two of furniture that you like can raise the quality of your life even in a place that you don't like very much.

The main change, though, needs to be in you. Don't try to ignore what you don't like and end up dissociating from the environment completely. Look for anything that you can appreciate. The way the sun shines through a particular window on a summer day, a winter view of rooftops covered in snow, or the way light changes during the day can all be little things to pay attention to.

Doing things to make where you live nicer doesn't mean that you're making a commitment to love something you don't. The commitment you're making is to yourself. You can treat yourself to good things, even if they are very small. Keeping up with chores because you believe you deserve to live in a clean home and can have nice surroundings is about giving yourself something good, even if life isn't lavishing things on you.

Althea's Story

"Mother always told me that a home was a reflection of the kind of person you are. She would say, 'If you have a messy house, you have a messy life.' I grew up in a house that was spotless. I can't stand a mess, but I also can't keep up, and I feel like I just want to scream when I come home and see the place. As much as I hate it, I stay as late as I can at work so I don't have to go home to everything that needs to get done."

Althea was in tears when she finished telling me about her dilemma. I asked her several questions to get a sense of just how terrible Althea's house was. Althea told me she hadn't made her bed in weeks and that her floors needed to be vacuumed. "Forget about dusting," she said. Then I asked her if there were things in her house that seemed unsanitary. Althea was shocked by the question. Of course there was nothing unsanitary. She just hated the messiness of the bed and the dust everywhere. Her mother would have been ashamed.

Althea valued seeing her friends, being productive at work, and cooking. She did not enjoy dusting and was often in a hurry in the morning, so she didn't take the time to make the bed. When she discussed all of this with me, she realized she didn't see the point in making the bed. This was her mother's thing, not her own. She stripped the bed and put on clean sheets once a week. She didn't mind that. It was a Saturday morning chore she did while listening to her favorite music. She also didn't care about dust, but she was plagued by the thought that she should make sure everything was dusted.

Especially when she was depressed, Althea thought that she was a disappointment to her mother—who had been dead for more than ten years. Althea recognized that she had made her mother's values and rules an obligation for herself, even though she didn't share them. She also recognized that her worries about disappointing her mother were not realistic. Wherever her mother was now, she surely offered enough grace to trust Althea with her own choices. Althea set a schedule for doing her various chores that allowed her to spend time on other things she valued. Yes, her house remained somewhat dusty, but she decided to let the dust be a "spiritual pact" between herself and her deceased mom. It was her way of reminding herself that it was okay to have her own rules and that she no longer had to follow someone else's rules for what her life should look like.

Living Well

- Staying on top of chores, home maintenance, car repairs, and bills is a lot for anyone. Fortunately, doing the laundry isn't an art and doesn't have to be treated like one. Give yourself some grace and go with "good enough."
- You may hold yourself to a standard that is exhausting, and it can be helpful to learn to tolerate a little mess in life. You can live your life now, even if things aren't perfect or you aren't in a situation that you particularly love. Doing little things to make your life nicer and staying on top of things so they don't build up and overwhelm you can help you live well.

6

interacting with others

Humans are social creatures. None of us can survive without the help of others. Whether your life is filled with many people or you're mostly alone, finding ways to interact positively—and to minimize negative interactions with difficult people—can help your mood. The strategies you've used earlier can also help when other people don't act in your favor. This chapter focuses on family, friends, and acquaintances. More intimate relationships will be covered in the next chapter.

Who's in Your Circle?

Because we all have private, inner worlds that other people aren't part of, it can sometimes feel as if we are alone. No matter how much you tell others, or how much you want to be understood, there will be limitations because nobody other than you can live inside your head. Likewise, no matter how much you know someone else, no matter how honest and revealing they are to you, they will always have a part of them that is private. And yet, it's also true that no one is truly alone. Whether we realize it or not, we all have other people in our lives, and it's important for our health to connect with kind and loving others.

To help you determine the various players in your life, fill out the Who's in My Life diagram. Consider the smallest inner circle, the bull's-eye, to represent the people who are most supportive to you. These can be close family or chosen family, a dear friend, or whoever you think of as having your back and being someone with whom you can share your true self. If you don't have such a person, think about someone you might like to get closer to; sometimes repairing a relationship is necessary so that a person you've become estranged from can be that center individual.

Some of the people who were in the innermost circle may no longer be in your life. This exercise is not intended to bring up sad memories or to cause you to dwell in grief. It's meant to account for who is currently here. Aim to list the people who are in your life right now. That said, feel free to list people from your past whose memories

WHO'S IN MY LIFE?

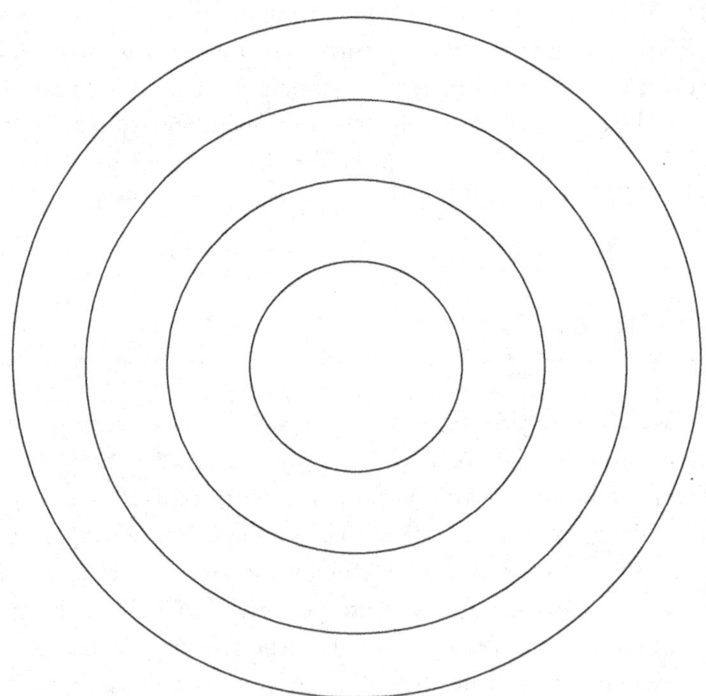

bring you joy. If you have had recent losses and this diagram task is too hard, put it aside for now, but don't avoid it altogether. Make a plan to return to it at another time.

In the next circle out from the center, you might list people you trust and with whom you enjoy spending time, with whom you may even share stresses in your life, but who would not be your closest confidants. You might have some family members with whom you have a solid relationship, who you can count on, but they aren't your closest relatives.

There is no pressure to fit people into the places in your life that you may have been socially influenced to think of as right or necessary. For example, Mom—or your own children—don't always need to be in the center, even if they are fine people who treat you well. Remember that you're considering what you value about relationships and who is most supportive. Let that be your guide, not the dictates of others.

As you move farther out, you might include friends with whom you have more limited contact. These may be people you don't speak with often, but when you have a conversation or get-together, it is like your friendship picks up where it left off. If you've moved around a lot, or if you've stayed in touch with a few people from college or high school, they may fit into this category. Coworkers and neighbors may be in this circle.

Keep moving out with the circles. You can even add more circles. For this exercise, you can even include familiar people you know through their jobs, like the barista you might say a few words to when you buy a coffee. More is better here. Think of as many people as you can. You might be surprised that you notice more possible support in your life than you thought.

You may be a relatively introverted person who enjoys your space, and you may not have a great need to be surrounded by people. Or you may tend to be more extroverted but currently feel like you don't have people in your life to rely on. Most people connect with a limited number of individuals and aren't always laughing and raising a glass in selfies. These social comparisons diminish the value we place on the many people we interact with as we go through the day. It's useful to define your social network, to think broadly about the people with whom you rub elbows regularly.

You may have people whom you would once have put in the circle, but, for some reason, no longer are there. Some people you may care about, but they create havoc in your life when you spend time with them. Write those names outside the circle or keep them out altogether. The point of this exercise is to take stock of where you find community—whether your life is still filled with close loved ones, or whether you need to make social connections by going to a store or café where familiar people work.

USE YOUR SUPPORT LIST TO CONNECT

Make a phone call, send an email, invite someone to take a walk during good weather. Don't get trapped in the idea that all conversations need to be deep to be meaningful; interact even with acquaintances in the outermost circles. A brief chat about the project you need batteries for with the employee at the hardware store can still be a positive connection with someone who can become part of the flow of your life. You may find it comforting to see a familiar face at places where you frequently run errands or with people at your gym—although customs about having conversations at gyms can vary.

If you wonder whether conversations need to be profound to be meaningful, try a small experiment. Innocuously eavesdrop on a conversation when you are out and about. What do you hear? Most people are likely talking about mundane, perhaps even boring things. And yet, their exchanges can still be a way to connect and lift the spirits.

Managing Your Social World Even When You Don't Feel Like It

Now that you've taken a look at who is in your life, it's time to examine how your thoughts, feelings, and actions can influence your connections. Thoughts and perceptions are not always in line with the facts of situations, especially when the gray-shaded glasses of depression may distort them.

Let's consider various common thoughts people with depression tend to have regarding their connections with others. Along the way, we'll consider strategies for thinking and acting differently so you can strengthen your social relations. Although the center of your concentric circles may not be biological family, as the physically closest group for many people, we'll begin there.

"My family doesn't understand me—what's up with that?"

Parents don't understand children, children don't understand parents, siblings disagree with one another, families have drastically different political views—isn't it all supposed to be easier? Well, no. Whatever kind of family you have, there will inevitably be stressful periods when you feel as though nobody understands you or wishes to do so. This is especially true during adolescence. For some lucky people, the time in our lives when we begin to assert a personality apart from family is met with support and curiosity by adult relatives, but for many it is met with strong resistance. If this has been the case for you, you may struggle with wanting to be understood.

Sadly, some of the interpersonal struggles within families don't run their course and everyone grows up and is okay with it. You might have left family years ago, but whenever there is a holiday, wedding, funeral, or other event that you attend—poof—you're instantly 12 years old again and the feelings of inadequacy, shame, anger, powerlessness, or any number of other uncomfortable emotions rise. Or perhaps your family has always been loving and supportive, but they don't understand your depression; you might even be asked, "What do you have to be depressed about?"

Negotiating family dynamics is complicated, and there are no one-size-fits-all solutions. If your experience is that you're misunderstood by family, you may have to accept that living well doesn't include a Hallmark moment of reconciliation, but it can reduce tension and distress, nevertheless.

ACCEPT YOUR FAMILY'S LIMITATIONS

A good place to start is with acceptance. There is a scene in the Holly Hunter movie *Home for the Holidays* in which Anne Bancroft's character says to her gay son, played by Robert Downey Jr., "You know me, I can't change," to which he replies, "Neither can I, Ma." You may find it hard to understand how the people in your family think and act the way they do, and you want to wake them up. It's quite possible that they can, in fact, change. Chances are, your desire for them to fit into your inner world will not be the impetus for them to change, though, because they also have their world that they want you to fit into. This is the dilemma. You want to be understood, they want to be understood—you're at loggerheads.

You don't need to agree with your family. Accepting them for who they are can be a good start. This doesn't mean trying to see their point of view when you find it to be inconsistent with your values. Accepting isn't acquiescing.

When the focus of your desire to be understood continues to end with your hurt and disappointment, you might turn the attention away from yourself. Consider that your family is doing what they can as a consequence of their learning history. When you adjust your expectations of them, it will be easier to tolerate the things you find annoying or hurtful. You might believe they should behave differently, but this *should* is another trap for you.

A demand that your loved ones should do one thing or another to remain close to you will likely be a demand that hurts you. It would be great if they saw your pain, celebrated your decisions, appreciated all you've done for them, but this may never happen. Your actions toward them are all you can control. What kind of parent, child, or sibling do you want to be? You can act according to your values even when others you care about cannot or will not share your values.

"Why can't I stop thinking I'm a terrible parent?"

You might believe that you don't deserve to receive understanding or empathy from your family. There is no reliable guidebook for parents, and the idea that everyone naturally becomes a good parent when children are born is a myth.

In your depressive state, you may have needed to turn all childcare responsibilities over to your partner. Perhaps you are a harsh disciplinarian or a softie who lets your children get away with more than you think is good for them. No matter what you believe you've done "wrong," there are strategies for checking facts about your thinking. For example, you can ask yourself, "Are you *really* such a horrible parent?" Probably not. "Can you do better?" Probably yes. The key is to assess whether your actions are in line with your values and adjust accordingly.

For example, you may take away your child's phone after seeing them make mean comments to someone on social media, and they scream, "I hate you!" But if you value kindness and believe that unkind actions should have negative consequences, you've acted in line with your values by taking away the phone for a period of time.

Believing that there is any one way a parent should be is a trap in this regard, like the other examples we've given of the problematic *shoulds*. Keeping in mind that we live here, now, you can only start here and move forward. Perhaps the damage done in the past is irreconcilable. In this case, the solution is to grieve and move forward. Expressing your sorrow but not expecting anything in return from children who you may have hurt is a good start. Then, practice kindness to others around you; building that habit will prepare you if your children or grandchildren seek a relationship in the future.

"Why don't my friends ever call me?"

I've heard this question so many times from so many of my clients over the years that I have come to believe that the ingredients to the answer are one part reality, one part perception, and one part shared negligence. Let me explain.

The *reality* may be that you get it in your mind to reach out to friends, and they don't do the same for you. It's possible that your friends have come to expect you to reach out to them. They have had nice conversations with you when you reached out, and then don't feel the need to stay in contact. You, however, may feel disrespected or abandoned by them.

The *perception* part is that some people may in fact reach out to you, but they aren't the people with whom you'd prefer to be engaging. For instance, your somewhat annoying neighbor may call you weekly, but you may not be registering those calls; you believe that nobody ever calls you, yet here's proof that you do receive calls. And you have to be the one to reach out.

The third ingredient, *shared negligence,* is acknowledging that avoidance may be happening on both sides of the phone call as you wait for the other to contact. This can lead to both parties thinking they always have to be the one to reach out or to feeling guilty that they haven't been more proactive. Rather than taking the reins and calling, both of you wait it out and feel sad.

CONSIDER THE MEANING YOU PLACE ON RECIPROCITY

When you have the thought that you always have to be the one to reach out to friends or family, what does that mean to you? Do you tend to believe that it means they don't care or don't love you? Do you feel judgmental toward them, as if they aren't doing their part? All of these beliefs are natural to have, but they are limited.

Thinking more flexibly, could you consider other possibilities? Maybe the person doesn't manage their time well and isn't organized enough to call regularly. Maybe they've gotten into the habit of expecting you to be the one who contacts. Perhaps they place other priorities first, and this is how they treat all of their friends and family. Or maybe they have cultural beliefs about people of a certain age being the ones to reach out, and you're in that age group. It's possible that they may be dealing with mental health issues that they don't want to disclose to you, and they may feel bad about not calling. These are not exhaustive reasons, and you may still find these reasons annoying or unacceptable.

Can you consider having a conversation without accusation, sharing your feelings and your perception that you're always the person reaching out?

MAKE THE BEST OF YOUR TIME ALONE

When you don't have a lot of contact with friends, you may feel lonely. However, being alone does not need to result in feeling lonely. Can you enjoy being alone and having the freedom to do what you like?

If you're forced to be alone for some reason, however, you might not enjoy it. You might be housebound because of an injury or an illness, and your time alone is not a choice. You may have moved far from people you know to take a job that will allow you to pay bills. Whatever your circumstances, if you find being alone to be a curse you desperately want to escape, and the fingers of loneliness are creeping up on you, you might be able to do some things to make the best of your time alone rather than experiencing it as hell. You might follow an interesting podcast, you could learn a hobby through YouTube tutorials, or simply read a good book. Even more simply, you could play background music that is either calming or allows you to tap your finger along with the beat.

SEEK OUT THOSE WHO SHARE YOUR INTERESTS

For most of us, it was easy to make friends at school, college, and the workplace.

What are your interests? What's important to you? You might find friends through those activities. This list of possible shared interests is by no means exhaustive, but it may give you some ideas that will suggest something you've not thought of before. Does anything else come to mind? If so, reach out to find like-minded folks.

- Book club
- Bible study
- Ball team
- Church
- Crochet group
- Camping group
- Dance class
- Distance learning online
- Hiking group
- Knitting circle
- Meditation center
- Mosque
- Quilting group

- Synagogue
- Volunteering for a political candidate
- Walking group

"What if I don't want to celebrate holidays with my family?"

Avoiding a family holiday may have too many long-term repercussions. Instead of bowing out altogether, you can set manageable boundaries. For example, maybe you only attend part of the event, such as going for dinner but not joining in a religious service, or meeting up after the main event.

When you're present at the family event, you may need to ensure you don't spend a lot of time in the same room as the relative that holds completely different political or religious views than you do. You might also be ready to change topics or end conversations if you have a relative that you know will bait you with their views. Focus on what you can enjoy: food, music, watching some of your favorite relatives laughing.

If you enjoy your family but believe you're too depressed to attend a holiday event, this can be an opportunity to practice getting out of your head and living in the moment. When you find your mind drifting to your own grim thoughts, look outward. Offer to help clean up the kitchen and do a task mindfully. Pay attention to what everyone is wearing and see how many people wear similar color clothing. Any of the things you pay attention to can also trigger negative thoughts. Simply bring your mind back to something to focus on outside of yourself; it may be as simple as noticing the changing shadows from the light entering the room as the day progresses.

LEAVE IF NECESSARY

You will always have the choice to leave. It's not a lie to say that you aren't feeling well if you can't beat the blues while you're trying to be with family. If it becomes clear to you that you can't think of conversations to start, or it feels unhealthy to engage with an annoying relative, you can use your own agency. Sometimes the healthiest thing to do is to walk away.

CREATE A FAMILY OF CHOICE

You may not have biological family with whom you engage, either by choice or by circumstance. When your family members are deceased, live far away, or are estranged, you can create your own family. You may have heard the expression, "You can choose your friends, but you can't choose your family." Indeed, that is true, but you can choose to make your friends your family. You can plan holiday celebrations with a small group of people whom you enjoy.

"What if I don't have any friends?"

Feeling like you're completely alone in the world might be a matter of perception like so many other things we've discussed in this book. You might be noticing only what or who you don't have and not seeing the people who do care about you. Avoidance can also be a bad habit here. Sometimes, especially if you've become isolated while you're depressed, you can continue to avoid contacting friends out of fear that they will be angry with you, or that they will not wish to be in touch after time has gone by. However, you might have the experience of contacting someone you've not spoken with for some time, and the two of you will be catching up and feeling like no time has gone by whatsoever.

Of course, some people with their own problems may respond with resentment or be upset that you weren't there for them. They may work this through with you, or you may need to allow that the friendship has ended. If you come to the realization that you were an unreliable or even nasty friend, you can take a few steps to amend the situation: 1. Apologize, 2. Seek forgiveness, 3. Grieve and move on, if the other person doesn't wish to rekindle a friendship. Then, seek out the company of others, start new relationships. Everyone can use a friend.

REFER TO YOUR SUPPORT CIRCLE

Look back at your support circle diagram. You might consider the people who are currently in the outer circles and consider how you might bring them closer to your center.

ENGAGE BRIEFLY

Here are a few simple ideas to help when you're feeling alone or lonely:

- Engage in brief interactions, and make opportunities to do so.
- Evaluate the judgmental thoughts that may follow, such as judging the exchange because you hadn't discussed anything profound.
- Don't talk only about your misery. People who care about you will want to know how you're doing, but few people can tolerate hearing only about bad things. Sometimes, when you're overwhelmed by misery, you might need to share that and then ask the other person what's going on for them.

"How can I spend time with my kids when I'm so depressed?"

You may be afraid you will pass on depression to your children, or if you have adult children, you might think you're being a burden on them. But consider this: If you had a broken arm and couldn't roughhouse with your children (kids or adults), you wouldn't avoid them altogether. You'd engage within your capacity. It's the same with depression. Here are a few tips:

- If you're avoiding young children by staying in your room and leaving childcare responsibilities to your partner, simply be present in the same room with them. You could even be playing a game on your phone or watching what they are doing, but don't isolate yourself.
- Find a low-stakes activity like sitting with your children and coloring in a book together. You don't have to pretend to be anything other than who you are, but you can use this to connect with your children and also as a mindfulness exercise.
- With adult children, call them on occasion. Ask them how they are doing. Take a walk with them. Keep the activity low-stakes.
- *Depressed thinking* styles might also get in your way. Those styles may be maximizing the negative or minimizing the positives of your relationship with your children; you may be succumbing to

those terrible *shoulds,* or you might believe that things are bad because you feel bad, but there may not be any evidence apart from the feeling.

"I'm so irritable, how could anyone stand me?"

No matter how angry you may be, know that you don't need to act on your feelings. The acting-from-the-outside-in suggestion here is also to act opposite an emotion that will cause harm in your relationships.

Before reacting, take a deep breath and slowly count to four as you exhale. Then calmly ask for a modification that would bring some relief. For example, if there's too much noise in your house, breathe deeply, then ask if the noise can be turned down a bit. This may also be a time to step away from the situation for a moment to another room, or out of the house.

You can also monitor and change your self-talk. When we are irritable, it's easy to tell ourselves we can't stand what others are doing, or that "they are so annoying I want to scream." Simply reminding yourself that tolerance is possible can help. You might say to yourself, "I would prefer they not do what they are doing, but I can stand it and I can cope with it." This can calm some of the irritability.

Living Well

- Act according to your values and work to set boundaries with others who may challenge your limits or ask you to do things that go against your values.
- The golden rule may sound trite, but "doing unto others" is what we can take charge of. What they do unto us, that's out of our control—but we can try to minimize the amount of hurt done to us by others.
- Keep in mind that you live in the present. Even if the past had some relationship upsets, you can reach out to people with whom you may

have lost touch and invite them to reconnect. Although you may have burned some bridges, you may also rekindle relationships that can be meaningful and support your living well.

- Slow down your reactions to others and your response to your own action urges. It helps you stay calm rather than attack others, or stay engaged rather than avoid the important people in your circle.

7

thriving with a partner

Relationships challenge everyone, but depression makes them even harder. Others may not understand the severity of your depression and respond in ways that invalidate your distress—for example, expressing frustration that you're distant or not more positive. The mood-induced unhelpful thinking and behaviors that pull you deeper into depression also push you away from others. However, what you've learned about thinking flexibly, acting in a values-driven fashion, and staying engaged in life applies equally to dating, relationships, and building satisfying lives with others.

This chapter isn't a guide for couples or a replacement for couples therapy. Research shows that when one or both partners live with depression, couples therapy may be the treatment of choice—something worth considering if you're currently in an intimate relationship. This chapter offers suggestions to help you maintain your relationship during difficult times. If you're not currently in a committed relationship, or if you've recently lost an intimate partner, you might skip this chapter. Doing so would be an example of *adaptive avoidance*—avoiding painful reminders that don't serve you well. You can return to this chapter when you begin dating again or enter an intimate relationship.

Viewing Your Relationship through a Narrow Lens

Thinking can undermine even our most intimate relationships. You might hold rigid beliefs about how your relationship should be. Such beliefs ruin relationships—the conviction that a spouse must behave a certain way, for example. Believing your partner should always be interested in what you have to say is unrealistic. Through a narrow lens, you may fixate on one aspect of a relationship (physical attraction, loyalty, fidelity) and ultimately sabotage it or prevent it from happening. Either you'll never find a perfectly stunning partner you fantasize about, or you'll believe your long-term relationship is over if you've lost some physical attraction to your partner. Consider what else is part of the relationship. You don't survive on bread alone, and a relationship built solely on sexual energy, absolute loyalty, or the belief you'll always see eye to eye is unlikely to last.

Viewing Your Relationship through a *Should* Lens

Setting ideals for a perfect relationship is another *should* trap. Many people remain alone because they haven't met their "ideal" person. They go on a date with someone who isn't tall enough by their standards, so they move on and look for someone else. Or the other person loudly smacks their lips while eating, which is irritating, so once again, they move on. There are endless differences—doesn't like sports, doesn't like the same music—so people never really get to know someone beyond such superficial characteristics. Ultimately, holding onto the belief that true love will meet all expectations may be a recipe for never finding it.

I've spent years working with people waiting for their ideal partner while living with terrible loneliness. This work taught me the importance of considering what's most meaningful to you about relationships.

Is it attraction or companionship? Is it having everything in common or having someone to come home to?

It's important to broaden what you find meaningful. You don't need to settle for someone who doesn't make you happy, but accepting another's imperfections can be valuable. You may not get everything in one package, but that doesn't mean the gift inside isn't good. The relationship you should have may never materialize.

People talk about finding a "soul mate"—a pleasant romantic notion, but there's no scientific, verifiable definition of what that is or how one would recognize it. Waiting for that "right one" may keep you doing exactly that—waiting. The implied definition of a soul mate is someone without imperfections who understands you completely. In other words, a unicorn.

Thriving with a Partner Even When You Don't Feel Like It

You can only work on yourself. If you start by trying to have a different relationship with your thoughts about relationships, or if you commit to acting consistently with your values rather than your *should* beliefs or idealistic imaginings, you might see a shift in your dating life or committed relationship.

Before offering general suggestions, one thing needs explicit clarification: While you can only change your own behavior, changing thoughts or actions should never put you in a subservient position, force a failing relationship to work, or make you settle for something that adds to your misery.

These suggestions that follow presuppose you're trying to make relationships work with others operating in good faith. You never need to change your behavior to please an abuser; the only required behavior change in that situation is finding a way to leave. You never need mental gymnastics to adopt someone else's beliefs when you don't share them. In short, work on yourself out of commitment to living well, not from forced appeasement of someone else.

Act as the Kind of Friend, Lover, or Partner You Value

All of the strategies we've referenced so far can help you act according to your values and in the way you'd like a friend, lover, or partner to treat you. Let's revisit a few strategies.

First, allowing your emotions (Chapter 1) helps you address, rather than avoid, concerns between you and your partner so annoyance doesn't fester into anger. Second, thinking flexibly (Chapter 3) lets you reconsider thoughts about your partner that may lead to assumptions, character assassination, or harboring negative thoughts about them. You can check the facts, reappraise your thoughts, or conduct behavioral experiments to confirm or disconfirm beliefs about your partner.

Finally, you can be proactive (Chapter 2) and act as if you're the kind of partner you want them to be, even when you don't feel like it. For example, if you're annoyed that your partner left the front door unlocked before bed, rather than yelling, you might lock the door and say, "I locked the door because it must have slipped your mind"—something innocuous.

Consider Mutually Setting the Rules

Many relationship types exist beyond the traditional heterosexual married-couple model of 1950s American television. You may think ground rules are silly, and for many intimate partners, tacit rules work fine. For others, however, not discussing what each person wants can result in false assumptions and hurt feelings. You can discuss all sorts of rules, including spending money, child-rearing responsibilities, household management, monogamy/nonmonogamy, guests staying over, family visits, holiday celebrations—the list goes on. Some couples allow considerable freedom but have "deal breakers" they cannot abide. For many, though not all, that's sexual infidelity. For many, though not as many as we'd like, any physical abuse is a deal breaker. Mutually setting rules or boundaries needn't result in a list of dos and don'ts, though if that's how you agree to do it, fine. It can be a loving conversation about what you're comfortable having a partner do and what would hurt too much. The conversation won't work if it becomes ultimatums like "If you ever cheat on me, you're out!" Rather, it's about having a real, non-confrontational discussion about the life you imagine and are willing to share with another person.

Look for the Softer Side

Sometimes we say things that consistently get under our partner's skin. After doing something you believe annoyed your partner, have you ever asked, "Are you mad at me?" and found it increased their annoyance? There's a common pattern couples therapists see called "demand/withdraw"[1] whereby one partner tries to engage and draw attention to something, and the other tries to retreat mentally or physically. Often this stems from different distress-management styles.

Some people need to talk things out so they "demand," and others need to calm down and center themselves before discussing, so they "withdraw." During times when neither of you is distressed, it helps to discuss how you each manage strong emotions. With mutual understanding, your interactions may be met with greater empathy.

"I'm unfulfilled in my partnership—but I stay anyway."

People stay in relationships for many reasons. Some rely on partners for financial security. Some don't want to disrupt their children's lives by separating. You might feel unfulfilled and unhappy but fear being alone, so you stay. When you don't want to leave but your relationship consistently fails to meet your needs, perhaps you can attend to your well-being in one or more of the following ways.

TALK ABOUT YOUR FEELINGS

It's hard to tell someone you don't feel fulfilled or aren't getting what you need from your relationship with them. You can make it easier for yourself as speaker and for your partner as listener by using active listening skills and "I" statements. Dr. John Gottman and colleagues have helped couples do this since the 1970s.[2]

When telling your partner about your feelings, use an "XYZ" formula: "When you do X, in Y situation, I feel Z." Notice there's no statement like "You make me feel Z." Here's an example: "When you said you'd be home by five last night in the snowstorm and didn't contact me until eight, I felt scared and worried." Saying this might be hard when you feel like saying, "Don't you ever do that to me again!!" The harsher statement feels relieving in the moment but won't improve your relationship long term.

When your partner responds, rather than immediately replying, pause and paraphrase what they said to ensure you understand them. This slows the conversation and keeps strong emotions under better control. Here's how this works, continuing the snowstorm example. Your partner says, "I thought I'd get out of work earlier but got held up talking to the boss, and then my phone was out of battery and I tried to get home as soon as I could."

You could reply, "So, you were trying to get out of work and be home by five, but you got held up and then wanted to get home as soon as you could, so you left but couldn't call from the car because your phone wasn't charged?" Could the partner have called from a work phone? Yes. Didn't the car have a phone charger? Probably. The point, however, is that the discussion can be slowed down so you can talk about your feelings and increase the likelihood of a commitment to interact differently in the future.

CONSIDER EXPECTATIONS

Sometimes we have ideals (similar to the *shoulds*) about what we want in a relationship and expect our partners to behave in certain ways. When they don't, we feel dissatisfied. If your ideal partner is a hopeless romantic who brings flowers and leaves love notes around the house, but you fell in love with a planner and problem-solver who takes charge of managing your lives, you may be disappointed by the lack of romance. In this example, the partner acts like an engineer, but you expect them to act like a poet. Ask yourself if your expectations about relationships might be unrealistic or unaccepting of your actual partner.

CONSIDER OTHER OPTIONS

You might never get everything you want from one person. Consider other ways to have your needs met. This should be openly discussed with your partner. Even something innocuous like wanting intellectual discussions and deciding to join a book club can impact the household; stating your need and planning ahead of time can lead to better understanding. It's more fraught to think about having sexual needs met through other options, but some couples do discuss open relationships. While this won't be acceptable for many people, it could be for some. This conversation may best occur with a counselor's help.

"I'm not really interested in sex—and feeling guilty about it."

For many, depression steals sexual desire. Low libido might be a symptom of depression or a side effect of necessary medication. Discuss this with a medical provider, but keep a few things in mind.

REMIND YOURSELF ABOUT WHAT'S TEMPORARY

Decreased sexual desire may change as your depression lifts. When you feel guilty that you lack interest when your partner has it, remind yourself this is part of a mental health condition you're living with. Would you feel guilty about not wanting sex if you had a raging fever and upset stomach?

Have a conversation with your partner that this isn't about them—if, indeed, it isn't. If you're willing and able to speak with a professional about it, let your partner know. Reassure yourself and your partner that this is a temporary situation. Just as your mood today doesn't predict your mood next week, month, or year, this is true of your low libido. It's a now thing, not necessarily a forever thing.

IDENTIFY WHAT'S IMPORTANT

For most, though not all, couples of every type, sex is important, regardless of age or relationship longevity. However, when you or your partner experience decreased desire, you don't need to discard the entire relationship.

LOOK FOR OTHER IMPORTANT ASPECTS OF RELATIONSHIPS

Can you enjoy intimate moments together that don't result in sexual activity? Spooning in bed or sitting in each other's arms while watching a streaming show can express love without pressure to perform. If you're feeling guilty because you don't feel like being sexual, can you offer to do something else important to your partner that you wouldn't usually want to do—like join them on a walk or accompany them to a play or a sporting event? Do you both value being good parents, and can you focus more on that shared experience?

"I still think about the one who got away . . . "

Sometimes current relationships are unfulfilling because we're haunted by a past relationship in which our hearts were broken, and we've set that individual up as the standard by which we compare all others. Perhaps you knew someone highly desirable was interested in you, but you didn't pursue it and now frequently fantasize about what it would have been like to be with them. This is a form of regret that's unhealthy and most likely inaccurate. Here's why.

LET GO OF THE PAST

We cannot change anything that no longer exists. You might think "the one who got away" is still out there, which may be true, but are they the same person you knew years ago? Would you still be interested if you actually had an opportunity to get together?

Some people used to love marshmallow fluff as children and get a craving to make a marshmallow and peanut butter sandwich as an adult—only to find they now think it's an unpleasant combination. Thinking we can re-create the past or pick up where we left off is never possible because we've changed, as have others around us. We only live in today.

CONSIDER HINDSIGHT BIAS

In Chapter 3 we introduced hindsight bias, or thinking there would have been a better outcome had we made a different choice or behaved differently in the past. This is biased thinking at work, when you can't stop thinking about a lost relationship. You remember being attracted and drawn to the person. If you never dated them, you remember them as an idealized portrait of who they were. Without knowing someone romantically and intimately, you only have your fantasy about what they would have been like, and you likely paint them as your Cinderella or Prince Charming.

In reality, they may actually be Nurse Ratched or a troll under a bridge. In your imagination they meet your needs, understand you always, don't have annoying habits, earn great money, have good taste—the list of their fabulous qualities could go on forever. In truth, they may be underemployed, lost in addiction, or have grown dumpier with age. When hindsight bias keeps you yearning for the one who got away, change your thought to allowing yourself to feel relieved that they were a catch and release.

BRING YOURSELF INTO THE PRESENT

In Chapter 6 we proposed engaging with others in a mindful way, paying particular attention to every aspect of the moment. *Mindfulness,* or being aware of present-moment sensations, can keep you in the present. Remember, all we have is now. This may feel like a radical step to take. Rather than going down the imaginary road not taken, focus on this moment. Even as you read this page. What is the shape of each letter? What shades of light surround you? Does your body feel light or heavy? If you're seated, do you notice the chair under you, feel yourself sinking into it? Are there scents in the air? Do you hear sounds—even subtle sounds, like soft ringing in your ears or the slight hum of an air vent? Let the past be the past and the future not yet be, and take this moment here, now.

> *"I'm unhappy, but as long as my partner isn't bothered, I don't bring it up."*

Your depression may be a response to an unhappy or untenable relationship. At the opening of this chapter, we discussed being the kind of partner you'd like to have, but doing so doesn't mean sacrificing yourself. Society puts considerable pressure on people, especially women, with statements like "Oh, she is a saint for staying with them." Holding up martyrs as heroes is well and good, but even if we never questioned the veracity of martyrology, those special individuals received some sort of mystical calling, and most of us never get such a nudge from the universe.

PUT YOURSELF FIRST

Being scared, miserable, or continuously angry in a relationship does no one any good. If you're keeping the status quo so nothing is disturbed for the children's sake, consider whether you're able to be your best self for them in your current situation. If you're accepting that your partner seems happy enough, so you don't want to rock the boat by sharing your feelings, you're likely not being your best self for your partner either.

Being your best self means taking a look at yourself. This may temporarily feel like selfishness. However, taking care of yourself doesn't equate to being self-absorbed. You need to put on protective gear before going into a burning building to save others.

CONSIDER THAT YOUR PARTNER MAY BE OPEN TO CHANGE

It's also possible your partner is keeping their own dissatisfaction or unhappiness to themselves because they believe you aren't bothered. Or, even if they're perfectly content, they may care enough about you to consider making changes that will be better for you. Keeping your feelings to yourself because you assume your partner doesn't need or want to change anything might be acting on inaccurate information. If it's difficult to bring up your unhappiness because it will be an unpleasant conversation, your silence is actually avoidance that may keep you free of momentary unpleasantness but unhappy in the long run.

END A BAD RELATIONSHIP FOR A GOOD OUTCOME

We tend to talk about breakups or divorces as failures. However, from a mental health perspective, a breakup or divorce handled in a manner that doesn't cause additional suffering to you or others is a success. In reality, sometimes the ending of a relationship is ugly, but that's not a reason to stay in a bad or unhappy relationship. If you've done all you believe you can do—and it may be wise to seek professional help—yet you're still unhappy, the answer may be ending the relationship, grieving, and moving forward.

If there are children involved, commit to working with your partner to make it as easy as possible for them. They likely have friends whose parents have split up. Maintain your own commitment to being the person you want to be and keeping your self-respect no matter how your partner behaves. Avoiding ending a relationship because it will hurt and be difficult might be the very thing maintaining your depression. You may look back and see that what you needed all along was a "partnerectomy."

Living Well

- Trying to force relationships into some ideal often results in loneliness or in making demands on those with whom you're intimate. This strains relationships. You can develop flexible approaches to relationships that allow you to have some needs met and to meet others' needs, even when it doesn't fulfill every hope or desire.
- Depression may complicate finding or maintaining a relationship. The strategies of being proactive, thinking flexibly, and allowing your emotions all can help within the context of intimate relationships. Living your life in the present, guided by your values, can help you take care of yourself, be a better partner or parent, or have a more fulfilling journey as a single person.

8

engaging with school, work, and hobbies

If you're in school or working full-time, a huge portion of your waking hours go to your studies or career. It's no surprise, then, that depression can have a significant impact in an area consuming so much of your time. How to handle it?

This chapter offers strategies—some covered earlier in different contexts—to help keep you engaged and productive at work or in school. The chapter also addresses re-engaging in activities you once enjoyed or trying new activities so you don't fall into the trap of "all work and no play." Overall, this chapter focuses on helping you find balance between the work you must do and activities that can provide restorative time.

School or work can eat up a lot of hours. The stresses of these activities can leave you feeling tired and overwhelmed. When you add depression on top of the stresses everyone experiences, you may feel paralyzed at work or school and believe you have no time for hobbies. However, having a combination of strategies to manage your depression—such as those presented in previous chapters—and developing strategies for setting achievable goals for work or school can be helpful. This chapter is not about time management or job hunting; it's about practicing setting and meeting goals and balancing all of this with pleasurable activities that can make life more satisfying than being a workaholic or studying all the time.

Effective Goal Setting

Most goals people have over their lifetimes concern work, school, or managing finances. Of course, these are all related. Goals you set for work include developing a certain career or finding a certain type of job. Some jobs will require some form of schooling, whether trade school, college, or an advanced degree. Ultimately, what you do for work will affect your resources and your finances.

Values, once again, play a role in the goals we set. You may value family over everything else and desire employment that allows ample time to spend with them. You may have a family with more than one income and can set different goals than if you were handling all the finances on your own. You might value prestige and will set goals to work toward a career that commands social respect. You may already be settled in your job or career but hope to achieve financial security. Start with what you value, what's important. When your goals, of any sort, align with your values, you're likely to be more satisfied.

Before going further, however, everyone starts at a different place, with different abilities and resources. The goals available to someone born into a wealthy family will be very different from those available to someone born into poverty.

Society is unequal and unfair, and you—simply because of your ethnicity, race, gender identity, or sexual orientation—will have additional stressors as you pursue goals. Or you may live in a part of the world where your work options are limited to factories or smaller businesses, like fast-food chains. Financial stress can create anxiety and distress. Your life may be such that you're trying to get through each day, and the idea of goals may seem like a lofty ideal that misses the point. We can think of goals as being very short term or long term, and sometimes they are immediate and based more on need than on desire. Either way, the suggestions that follow will help you set and stick to goals, even when depression clouds your motivation or sense of hope.

Engaging with School, Work, and Hobbies Even When You Don't Feel Like It

Pleasurable activities are an excellent counterbalance to the must-do labor of careers and school. Tap into your values (discussed in Chapter 4) to find what matters to you in leisure, and make those things part of a routine. Planning something enjoyable at the end of the day helps you resist less helpful ways of coping with work or school stress. Planning to spend time playing a board game with your kids and following through on that plan after a rough day will likely be better than having a stiff drink when you get home.

A definitive break between work and leisure also helps. Whether you have the kind of job you can leave behind at the end of the day, or you routinely take work home, set aside time to disengage from work, to rest your mind and avoid burning out. Sometimes we have to bring work home, stay late, or work overtime. It's not possible to be a student only when you're in class. The COVID-19 pandemic gave people around the world the experience of their homes becoming their place of work and school, which made it more difficult to get away from stressors.

Having a plan for something that brings your mind into the present and separates work from leisure—like spending 30 minutes with your favorite music or sitting down to a cup of tea—can help. If you have limited time, perhaps even taking a quick shower and focusing on the feel of the water can mark the shift from obligation to personal time and help you recharge for the next day.

"I'll never get the job I want. Why even try?"

While this thought may seem reasonable, it's an example of inflexible thinking discussed in Chapter 3. Let's break this down. When you think something will never happen, you're fortune-telling. You may rightly know that something is improbable, but improbable is not the same as impossible. Even if there aren't options immediately available to you, that doesn't mean opportunities won't present themselves. That hopeless question—"Why try?"—inadvertently works to make your prediction come true. If you don't look for what's out there, you won't see opportunities.

Sometimes, though, we hope to find our dream job—or our passion. This type of goal can come with a level of privilege you may not have, unfortunately. For example, if your only local employment opportunities are in manufacturing or farming, and your passion is to be an artist, but you aren't creating anything and there are few opportunities to practice, this passion is mostly fantasy. People who have their basic needs met can pursue "passions"; you may be trying to get your footing. This doesn't mean you should give up hope of finding work that is closer to what you want to do.

We also don't know what any job or career will be like until we're in it. So often people say things like "My passion is for X," and then when they find work in that field, they recognize that everything has upsides and downsides. Don't give up—but recognize that there's no perfect future, and it's wise to live well now. Keep looking for options that can change your life.

CHECK THE FACTS

Thinking more flexibly about work or school can start with checking the facts. When you believe you will never have the job or career you want, and that it's not worth trying, start by looking at what's available to you. You may be more qualified than you think, or ready to do things you couldn't before.

When you were younger, you may have been told that you didn't have good enough skills, and that's why you did poorly in a particular class or weren't chosen to help your parents with a special task. That belief may simply be outdated.

There may also be help available to you now that was not when you were younger. For example, sometimes people have difficulties in school when they're young. The difficulty may be due to undiagnosed learning problems that went unnoticed by busy public school personnel. As an adult, you might look into services that are available at colleges and universities for accommodations that could assist your success.

If you feel stuck in a current work situation and are worried that you don't have the proper education or training, or that you've not been good at learning new things, you may still be seeing yourself inaccurately. Many people return to school as adults, when they're ready to focus on their studies, and start at a local community college. Being ready often translates to doing well, opening doors to the next step in your education.

Look at job possibilities that attract you; they may be good fits for you. But first you have to take the leap and apply. You may think you're not qualified for a certain job because of the prerequisites listed. But keep in mind that some prerequisites are preferred rather than required; seek out jobs with preferred prerequisites. When depression is coloring your thinking, you might ignore job openings because you interpret preferred skills you don't have as signs you won't succeed. But that's not certain. It never hurts to inquire before ruling yourself out—you may have exactly what employers are looking for but don't trust yourself yet.

SET SMART GOALS

Goals need to be specific, measurable, attainable, relevant, and time-limited (SMART).[1] When it comes to finding a job you want, being specific with a goal may start with something like "Review websites for employment opportunities with companies that interest me. I'll review two listings per day for a week." Maybe your SMART goal can be to update a résumé or curriculum vitae, or complete an online job application. Make your goal achievable and relevant for you, and relatively immediate and short term.

BE THE ACTION NOW THAT YOU DESIRE IN THE FUTURE

Maybe you believe you won't get the job you want, and you say to yourself, "I'll never find the job I want, so why try? But if I could get this job, I would finally have what I want. I'd be happy. I could enjoy myself and I wouldn't be so frustrated all the time." According to acceptance and commitment therapy, these thoughts keep you disengaged from today and waiting to begin your life once something happens that will change everything.

However, your opportunity to live is now, so even when you're setting a goal to pursue further education or to find a preferred job, you can find what's available and important to you now, and live today—not in a hoped-for future. For example, you don't need a college degree to read on a topic of interest—you can explore on your own. Or, if you need to work an extra job, like delivering food, you might play particularly enjoyable music in your car, or take a pet along for the ride, or take a moment to meet new people. Finding ways to enjoy your life now does not preclude working on goals for the future.

"Sometimes I don't feel like showing up to work or school."

The times when you don't feel like showing up are when working from the outside in becomes useful. Feelings are mercurial, and they come and go. When you're depressed, the pull is likely toward doing little, especially when paired with a belief that you can't show up. Fears that you might fail can also make you not want to do things.

The steps to working from the outside in (see Chapter 1) offer ideas you can try when you aren't feeling it. Recall that the ARC of emotion has three parts: the emotion, the thoughts, and the action urge. Here the emotion may feel more like a dullness or lethargy. The thought may be along the lines of what the British say: "I just can't be asked." The action urge may be not to go to work, an interview, or class.

Instead, take some action; for example, contact your employer and request personal time off, or reschedule an interview. See if you can get lecture notes if you miss a class. You may not succeed from the "outside"—to go wherever you need to be—but you can still partially show up and take a step toward acting on a goal rather than a feeling.

CREATE A SCHEDULE

When the task ahead of you is something you do regularly, instead of listening to your emotions, listen to your calendar. Plan some time each week to work on tasks. Plan to read some of your assignments each day or go into work and take small steps toward completing the tasks you need to do. For example, if you work at a grocery store checkout, it may be difficult to plan small steps—the items will keep coming on the conveyor. However, you can set a small goal to greet each customer and smile at them when you scan their rewards card or hand them a receipt.

RECOGNIZE MAGICAL THINKING

Not engaging while telling yourself that everything will work out is *magical thinking.* You won't pass an exam if you don't study. You won't keep your job if you're continually late or miss too many days of work.

This is also true of the belief that "it doesn't matter." Although we don't often see this statement as magical thinking, in a way, it is. While it may be a thought that stems from hopelessness, it *will* matter. There are consequences to action and inaction. Either everything will stay the same, which isn't good if you're feeling low and can't be bothered, or the change will be something undesirable, like getting a poor grade or being fired. Don't let your mind fool you.

"I hate this job, but I can't imagine leaving."

Depression may be coloring every aspect of your work life, which is why looking for what's good about where you work matters—it may lessen your desire to leave. Additionally, you may not be able to imagine leaving a job—or any situation—you're genuinely unhappy without of fear or self-doubt. Taking some small steps to celebrate even little successes can slowly build confidence. Finally, you might not imagine anything different because you don't know what else to do. There might be more available to you than you know, or it may be that the job that is bringing you down needs to take second place in your life.

LOOK FOR OPTIONS

When trying to solve problems, it's best to consider as many possibilities as you can. The technique of brainstorming is to throw out ideas; some people refer to this as spitballing. In other words, it's tossing out everything that comes into your mind. You may ultimately decide that some ideas are ridiculous, but don't judge them initially. Let your thoughts run away with ideas. This process can open up things you may never have considered, and it might spark a plan for leaving a bad job.

Once you have a list of ideas, you can consider the pros and cons of each, and delete ideas you would never pursue. Winning the lottery, for example, is always a great answer for getting out of a rotten job, but when you consider the pros and cons of continually spending money with such poor odds, it might be something you take off a list of feasible options. Make a plan for looking into potential opportunities. The goal is to find a way to make a change that can possibly improve your life.

MAKE YOUR LIFE OUTSIDE OF WORK PRIMARY

Whether you "hate" your job only on certain days, such as when many annoying things happen, or you have a job that is generally good but not your ideal, you might need to prioritize your life outside work. When you have a career that has become your identity, this might be particularly difficult, but it's still necessary. Remember, you were "you" before you became the title on your name tag. Try to connect with people who knew you from earlier in your life and might help you to consider that your work life and profession aren't everything.

Short-term, immediate goals can also help you live now and prioritize your life outside of work. When you're home after a day's work, what calls for your attention? Is it playing with the dog? Spending time with your kids? Preparing a meal? Sleeping? All of these activities can be interrupted by worries about work or school, rehashing a bad experience, or feeling down about a lackluster situation.

You can redirect your thinking. For example, if you're walking the dog and your mind drifts toward work, remind yourself that your immediate goal is to walk the dog and that's all that matters right now. You can't do anything about work while walking; you can make sure the dog doesn't get in other people's way. Watch your dog sniffing around or bouncing when it walks. Does this sound like attention to experience? Yes, exactly. Attend to the immediate goal and make showing up for your life outside work your main aim.

"I lost my job, and I'm too overwhelmed to look for another job."

Losing a job, no matter the reason, is demoralizing and frightening. Jobs provide a sense of stability and sometimes even community. When that is taken away, you can be left with uncertainty. Often, there's no easy or immediate way to secure another job. Some people apply repeatedly and still don't get hired. Consider what you can control in this situation.

GIVE YOURSELF A BREAK

Start by getting rid of self-blame. Whether you were fired because of something you did or didn't do, laid off because of the company's finances, or a business folded, punishing yourself with recriminations won't fix the situation or help you find one. Self-blame will feed your depression.

Severing ties with your employer can hurt. As the saying goes, "It isn't personal, it's business." However, it will feel very personal! What you need during a time like this is a little grace. Allow yourself the space to feel sad or angry. When those emotions come up, don't immediately shut them down. Remember that you don't need to engage in any action—and probably shouldn't when you're going through an unstable time.

FIND ASSISTANCE WHEN AVAILABLE

Social supports exist when you're out of work—but you'll need to take steps to access them. Unfortunately, we—ourselves and others—can judge those receiving unemployment benefits or food assistance.

If you've never needed to before, you might feel ashamed to go to a food bank. Yet, seeking assistance may be the immediate goal that will help you. Unhelpful thinking, such as *personalization*—the thought distortion of believing you're a bad person—can be countered by facing the full context. See the facts: You're out of work, you need to eat, you can do what you can to find work, and in the meantime, use the services available to you—you have a right to them.

WORK ON YOUR RÉSUMÉ

Following the principle of taking small actions that are likely to guarantee success, make updating your résumé something you get done (see Chapter 5). Start by adding your most recent job to the résumé. If that's all you can handle, set it aside, then return to make sure your personal details, like your address and phone number, are current. Do one thing to your résumé each day. These are small steps that get you closer to securing employment.

SET A SCHEDULE FOR LOOKING FOR JOBS

It's true that looking for a job can be a full-time job. To avoid burnout, it might not be helpful to search for eight hours a day, five days a week. But having some regularity can keep you moving forward. Use an activity chart (see Chapter 2) to schedule times when you will research jobs, fill out applications, or follow up on leads. Doing this for an hour two or three times per week according to the schedule can become something you do automatically.

Of course, there is an emotional toll in sending out applications and either not getting responses or being turned down for positions. The former feels like an insult after you do the work of completing an application and hearing no reply, and the latter feels like a kick in the gut when you aren't offered a job. It may take a combination of all the strategies discussed so far to help you manage disappointment on top of depression. To recap, you can have a different relationship to your thoughts and recognize when your thoughts are unhelpful. You can use skills to think more flexibly, act from the outside in, and engage in activities that can offer some relief from the stressors of job hunting. Finally, reach out to your social supports.

"I avoid my boss or my professors."

When job or school responsibilities have fallen by the wayside during a time of depression, you might not feel like facing a boss, professor, or advisor. If you're in this position, managing thoughts, feelings, and behaviors can help you get back on track. Approaching the person you're avoiding will, in the long run, be better than staying out of touch indefinitely.

Two kinds of unhelpful thinking (discussed in Chapter 3) often fuel the desire to avoid an authority figure after a long absence. The first is *fortune-telling:* Your continued avoidance amounts to a negative prediction you likely can't support. The second is *catastrophizing*—expecting the worst.

REMEMBER THAT A GOOD OUTCOME IS EQUALLY LIKELY

An alternative to catastrophizing and fortune-telling is to stay open to the reality that you don't know what the person's response to you will be. Even if the person is annoyed with or disappointed in you, they may also have some empathy. Usually, a boss or particularly a mentor or academic advisor will be relieved to hear that their employee or student is okay; they'll likely even help find ways to catch up on any work you've missed.

We can't predict the future, so remain open to all possibilities. Even if you have a catastrophic prediction, remember that a good outcome is equally likely.

ACCEPT IMPERFECTIONS

You might be staying out of contact with a boss, supervisor, or advisor because you aren't satisfied with the amount or quality of work you've completed. You may be dreading their reaction if you haven't done the best you can. You might not have made any progress and are avoiding owning up to that.

The person evaluating your work may be a perfectionist. That doesn't mean you have to be one too. Let them comment and micromanage your work, if that is their job. You may find it annoying, but if they are picky, that is their characteristic; it says very little about you and more about their personality. If you're getting work completed and you're doing the best you can, accept the comments, implement corrections, and keep handing in work that is less than perfect. If you're told specific details that need attention, follow through, but the main goal is to show that you're still endeavoring to meet expectations.

DEAL WITH THE DISAPPOINTMENT OF OTHERS

You may never fully meet others' expectations. Their expectations may be too high, as is the case with the perfectionist supervisor. Or you may not be as good at certain aspects of your work as others would like you to be. Not every good employee is fast with numbers; not every student is a great writer. When other people are disappointed in you and you're depressed, you might experience this as a weighty burden that feels as if it could break you. Their disappointment gets turned into you being the disappointment.

When someone is disappointed in your work, does that trigger unhelpful or depressive thinking? One common type of "distorted" thought that pops up in response is to overgeneralize; you may have disappointed someone this one time, but you tell yourself that you *always* disappoint *everyone*. Another is personalization; you may believe that *you* are a disappointment, as if it were a personality trait. Look at the evidence both for and against this belief. You'll find the truth is more balanced.

"I don't participate in any of the things I used to like to do."

Anhedonia, or not experiencing pleasure, is a common symptom of depression. You may not participate in activities you once enjoyed because they don't bring the pleasure they once did. You may wonder, "How can pleasant activities be a counterbalance when I don't find anything that gives me pleasure?" This is a reasonable question. You might need to approach the activities that once gave you pleasure and accept that, for right now, they will be, well, *meh*.

Instead, choose activities that are more likely to have elements of sensuous pleasure, like stroking a pet's fur or soaking in a warm bath. Pay attention to the softness of the fur or to the warmth on your skin. In the tub, use fragrances you can tolerate to improve the experience, like bath oil beads or a scented candle. Meditate on the scent.

LET GO OF THE OUTCOME

Has this ever happened: You've been eating the same pizza parlor pizza for a while, and no matter how much you like it, you realize you'll never regain the taste of your first slice in quite the same way? A similar thing can happen with activities we used to enjoy. You may feel somewhat numb to the activity, or you may feel tormented because you remember when the activities were enjoyable or even exciting. Charles Schulz depicted this experience with the character Charlie Brown. Charlie knew that he "should be happy" that Christmas was coming, but he wasn't.

Thinking about how you should feel—or once felt—steals even more pleasure from the moment. Instead, engage in the activities that fit with your values and worry less about whether they once felt better. Over time, you may find that you actually take some pleasure in things when you least expect to.

Living Well

- Much of life is spent working. To stay engaged with necessary tasks when you're depressed, recognizing and changing unhelpful thoughts and behaviors is a good starting point. Setting SMART goals sets you up for success. No matter how down you're feeling, you can still accomplish one small step.
- Avoidance of cumbersome activities or of people in authority will likely make things worse. Find ways to approach rather than avoid. Use an activity schedule to assign times to work on tedious tasks. Set a time limit so you don't feel as if your entire day is one long arduous slog. Reach out to a boss or instructor and talk through how to refocus on what they expect from you.
- If others are critical of you, do your best and accept their disappointment, but don't accept their judgment of you as a person. Not getting work done, or doing a less-than-perfect job, may merit a correction or critique, but it does not make a statement about you as a human being.
- Work–play balance is integral to well-being. But it's easy to forget, so we may need reminders. Adding leisure activities is important even when they may not bring the kind of pleasure they did prior to your being depressed.

9

considering what's greater than you

Life is not only about work deadlines, getting an education, housework, or maintaining relationships. These are all very important aspects of life, but other concerns may be weighing more heavily on you, particularly when you're depressed. Questions regarding the purpose or meaning of life may run through your mind. You may ask yourself, "Why does it all matter?"

People arrive at answers in different ways. We'll look at an approachable sampling of ideas from philosophy and theology that might help you when you wrestle with larger-than-life questions.

Looking to Something Bigger than Yourself

While the data is not altogether without contradiction, some research suggests that people who are more altruistic are less vulnerable to depression. Other research suggests that volunteering or helping others may have beneficial effects for people with depression, although the exact causal connection is not firmly established.

The therapeutic literature, especially that written by practitioners of acceptance and commitment therapy (ACT), emphasizes the importance of understanding one's values—what's important to you in your life—and acting consistently with your values (see Introduction and Chapter 1). Thinking about your values is more ephemeral than thinking about what you'll do on a Saturday afternoon. Identifying your values brings you closer to answering *why* questions, although not completely. There aren't easy answers to life's big questions, which is why even adults can be somewhat like toddlers, asking why repeatedly.

Rather than asking why, which often leads to another question, consider two options: One is to act as if the big questions have answers. For example, you might believe that life is existentially meaningless but live as if there is important meaning in everything you do; another example is to disbelieve in any kind of rule-giving deity or deities but live as if there is a moral being that desires you to live in a certain way.

The second option is to look beyond yourself. You can look to a "higher power" to help you through life's trials. Or you can see yourself as one being in a long history of human existence, taking your focus off your immediate life and feeling less isolated in your struggles.

Spirituality

People have different notions of religion or spirituality, and vary in the importance they place on it in their lives. You may be a highly religious person, or you may consider yourself spiritual but not religious; either way, your depression may seem confusing and at odds with your beliefs. Or, you may think, "Spiritual, schmiritual" and consider yourself a steadfast empiricist with no room for belief in higher powers. And yet, feeling confined by depression, pulling you inward, can feel like a continual downward spiral. Looking outward, to something bigger—whether a god or the planet on which you live—opens you up to move beyond that confinement.

"Religion," "spirit," and "the sacred" are all words that psychologists seldom write about. Yet, living well with depression means finding peace with larger life questions rooted in these topics. Most of the philosophies throughout recorded history have some form of emphasis on freedom from the self. In ancient Hindu and Buddhist thought, this is often attained through ritual practice or meditation, and followers in these traditions seek enlightenment.

Nearly all the religious traditions in the world, theistic or atheistic, emphasize the requirement to be kind to others or to all creatures. Of course, operationalizing kindness varies not only in religious tenets but also among individuals. Some people believe it's a kindness to save others from themselves by controlling their behavior, whereas others see this type of control as inherently unkind and believe operational kindness is doing good to others.

While many people connect with others and find meaning in life through religious communities, humanists do not consider a need for gods or a spiritual world in order to look outside of themselves. Child psychologist and author Nasser Yousefi writes in *The Humanist* about growing up during the Iraq–Iran war and not liking people, particularly adults.[1] He was depressed during his university years. But then he turned his attention to many humanitarian efforts, particularly working with children from remote villages in many different nations. He reports that, over time, he felt happier and that it was healing to work with people.

Our Common Humanity

You may agree that helping other people is a good thing, and it may make you feel even more isolated when you don't have the wherewithal to do so, or to connect with a community of helpers. You may, understandably, question why you struggle with depression when other people seem to go through life without this same struggle, making you feel alone, perhaps even embittered.

During the height of the AIDS epidemic in the United States, as I worked with many clients living with the illness, I would frequently hear "This should never happen." While I completely agreed that the suffering at that time was a terrible thing, I saw that people could take some solace knowing that there have been various plagues in human history; what was happening in the late 20th century had happened in some fashion in centuries past. It all felt less personal and less punishing, and gave people a connection to a common humanity.

Admittedly, knowing that others have suffered does not make the suffering easier. Just because there's a long history of people enduring torturous deaths by fire and sword doesn't make one excited to go to the stake. While Aristotle believed that suffering could be a source of character development, others, like Nietzsche, believed there was no meaning in suffering.

The enduring experience of depression can feel qualitatively different from other forms of suffering. Still, recognizing that you're not completely alone, that others share and have shared this experience, may provide some solace. This is a basic premise of group therapy and self-help groups; having a shared experience with others can provide support. Not everyone finds engaging in such groups beneficial, but perhaps it's enough to know you're not alone.

Considering What's Greater than You Even When You Don't Feel Like It

"My life has no meaning or purpose."

You don't need religion to find meaning. You don't need to make a huge impact on the world. Knowing what's important to you allows you to be the kind of person you want to be and to act accordingly.

REVISIT YOUR VALUES

Your values may not answer the big questions of existence, and they may not provide an ultimate meaning. However, each of us has a brief time on Earth, and within our particular circumstances we can engage in values-driven behavior. It doesn't require money or even great health to say a kind word if you value kindness. If you value family, sending a quick note to a relative to make a connection takes only a minute of your time. You may value success yet have faced great disappointments; in this case, perhaps you can redefine what success means to you and work toward doing something that can provide you with a sense of accomplishment, no matter how small.

"Why me?"

Most people hold an implicit belief that the world is just, and that good things happen to good people and bad things to bad people. When you're depressed and have been trying to live with it for some time, a belief in a just world is challenged.

Do your struggles with depression mean you're a bad person? Are you supposed to find something good in the midst of this all? If you're a person who holds religious beliefs, you may also struggle with your depression challenging those beliefs. In his book *When Bad Things Happen to Good People,* Rabbi Harold Kushner writes, "The idea that God gives people what they deserve, that our misdeeds cause our misfortune, is a neat and attractive solution to the problem of evil at several levels, but it has a number of serious limitations."[2]

CONSIDER THAT WHY ISN'T THE QUESTION

Perhaps we can all take a lesson from the author Kurt Vonnegut Jr., who, in his novel *Slaughterhouse-Five,* wrote this dialogue as the main character entered a flying saucer:

"Billy licked his lips, thought a while, inquired at last: 'Why me?'

'That is a very *Earthling* question to ask, Mr. Pilgrim. Why *you?* Why *us* for that matter? Why *anything?* Because this moment simply *is* . . . ' "[3]

ASK "WHY NOT ME?"

Consider asking yourself, "Why not me?" rather than wondering why something bad has happened to you. Only a small percentage of people living today and throughout history attain great wealth, have perfect health, achieve everything they work for. The majority of talented artists, musicians, and actors never achieve fame, no matter how gifted they are. As another example, many very intelligent people across our globe do not have the opportunity for advanced education.

Consider that less than one percent of people worldwide have a net worth over one million U.S. dollars.[4] Approximately the same number of people worldwide have two different color eyes.[5] Both are extremely rare. Looking at what's most common, roughly 40 percent of people on Earth have a net worth less than one hundred thousand U.S. dollars (or its equivalent).[6] Put into perspective, a substantial portion of humans do not have financial wealth, fame, or outstanding success.

Furthermore, regardless of our monetary status, we are all susceptible to physical and mental illness, unhappy relationships, addiction, and dissatisfaction with life. Knowing that we are all frail humans and that bad things happen, you may feel less alone in whatever difficulties you're going through. Millions of your fellow humans are in some type of distress, and at a basic level, we are all in this together.

"Has God abandoned me? Am I being punished?"

This fear is similar to the question "Why me?" You may feel insignificant and fragile, and wonder what you did to deserve having to live with depression. You may feel troubled by the worry that you did something to bring this sadness upon yourself. If you believe that God is punishing you, then you must believe there is a God or that there is someone or something to do the punishing. Every major theistic religion teaches that God is always with you and that God forgives.

LOOK AT SACRED TEXTS

Approximately 5.9 billion people identify with Judaism, Christianity, or Islam. The writings considered holy scripture in all of them speak of a loving and forgiving God. The Hebrew scriptures repeatedly state that God's steadfast love endures forever.

In the Christian Bible, the Apostle Paul says in Romans 8:38–39, "For I am sure that neither death, nor life, nor angels, nor principalities, nor things present, nor things to come, nor powers, nor height, nor depth, nor anything else in all creation, will be able to separate us from the love of God in Christ Jesus our Lord." This sounds rather comprehensive. The Quran 25:70 states that "Ever is Allah forgiving and merciful."

Hinduism, with 1.2 billion followers worldwide, recognizes in most of its sacred writings that actions have consequences that must be dealt with, and that forgiveness is available.

Consider what we might conclude from all of this: If you believe in a deity or deities, the evidence suggests you can find connection and comfort when you seek it, and that the deities are not inclined to abandon you.

Where does this leave the approximately 3.6 billion people on the planet who don't identify with these religious beliefs? Nihilists believe there is no inherent meaning in life. Existentialists believe that there is no meaning in the world apart from that which we as rational beings make. Absurdists believe there is no inherent meaning, yet maintain that we can accept this without being defeated by it. None of these philosophies leads inevitably to despair.

"Will this grief ever end?"

The singer Jim Morrison famously shouted "No one here gets out alive" at one of his concerts. A truer statement was never made, although thankfully not about that particular Doors performance. If you live, you face loss. Although customs vary in how people do it around the world, everyone grieves at some point in life. Grief is not depression, although they can feel similar. Grief is longing for something, or especially someone, whom we love or rely on. Usually, grief is shorter-lived than depression—although apart from cultural expectations regarding appropriate expressions of grief, there is no right or wrong way or set timeframe. When we grieve, we think about what we have lost; we may cry or wail; we may sit in silence.

REMEMBER THAT GRIEF IS TEMPORARY

While you may always miss a deceased parent, child, spouse, or even a beloved pet, the intense anguish of initial grief will not continue unabated. Life takes over and you move forward. Some people fear this because they believe that when the hurt subsides they lose their loyalty to the one they've lost. However, your love or devotion to someone cannot be measured by a formula that equates suffering with depth of love.

Or you might fear the opposite—that if you let yourself fully experience the sorrow, you will be stuck in this spot forever. Leaning into the pain, letting the memories come, sitting with old letters or photographs, while intensely difficult in the moment, can actually help you to incorporate the loss into your continued existence. A traditional Jewish expression to comfort the bereaved is "May their memory be for you a blessing." Yes, you may have moments when the grief feels fresh even years after a loss, particularly on a birthday or holiday, but it passes. Let it remind you of what you shared with another person in your life.

"How can I not be afraid to die?"

I was asked this question once as I sat at the bedside of a man in hospice. The patient's physician had asked me to visit and help the patient manage his anxiety, as it was not medically safe to give him higher doses of antianxiety medications. The patient had also refused to meet with any religiously affiliated chaplain or clergy member.

Admittedly, my training in treating anxiety and depression was not sufficient to give me an answer for a dying man gripped by fear. I had to admit that being afraid to die was very human, and that I shared the fear. What I could do in that moment was change our focus. Since neither of us could look ahead with any certainty to what awaited him, we could review what he knew. I asked him to tell me about his life, any stories he wished to share.

The late senator and former prisoner of war John McCain considered courage to be acting in the midst of fear rather than the absence of fear. Fear of death is ingrained in all sentient beings. Without it, species would not have survived. A small mouse fleeing a looming hawk may not be thinking "I don't want to die!" but it has an instinct to run, hide, and avoid being eaten.

You can face your own mortality with courage while being afraid. Continue to try to be your best self, and this best self may at times be irritable and short-tempered, or crying out for relief. Grasp a hand held out to you, think about the story of your life, whether you'd consider it a comedy, drama, or tragedy. Allow yourself to fear the unknown. Seek comfort from the people whose ministrations you welcome.

"What if I want to die?"

When you're living with depression, you may have thoughts of taking your life. Every person is capable of taking their own life—that is a reality. So why not do it? First, when you contemplate ending your life during a time of distress, you're likely feeling that your anguish will never end and that death is the only way out. But as we've discussed, moods change. What feels unbearable in this moment will likely not feel as deeply painful in time.

The story of Odysseus in Homer's *Odyssey* tying himself to the mast of his ship so he could hear the song of the Sirens has frequently been used as a metaphor for protecting yourself when suicide seems like your only relief. In the story, the Sirens sang so beautifully that passing ships would steer toward them, only to be destroyed upon the rocks. To avoid destruction while still hearing their song, Odysseus had his crew put wax in their ears so they would not be drawn by the singing. Then he ordered them to tie him to the mast so that he could hear the singing and not steer toward destruction despite the allure of the Sirens.

Find a way to keep yourself safe even though the strong pull of suicide may be present—stay with a friend or family member, seek professional help, go to a hospital to keep yourself "tied to the mast" until the crisis has passed. A list of suggested resources and readings specific to helping you when you're thinking of harming yourself can be found at the companion website for this book, *www.guilford.com/martell3-materials.* You may not see any other way out now, yet alternatives exist. You may think that you'll never escape this dark place. Our common humanity matters here too—millions of others have been in the same mental place and stayed alive, even when their pain was unbearable, ultimately experiencing profound change and regaining the desire to live.

Aging and Depression

As you get older, you have more life experience behind you to help you weather challenges, and you also face more change and loss. Behavioral activation, acting from the outside in, has proved helpful for many people dealing with depressed mood related to aging. Don't be tripped up by the word "act" here. Certainly, you can take up a hobby or volunteer, but acting can also mean pursuing a simple activity like looking through old photos and reminiscing. You might take a brief walk outdoors if you're physically able, or simply open a window and breathe in fresh air. Although you might feel like staying in bed (the pull from the inside), you can set an alarm and wake in time to enjoy a sunrise.

An ancient Sanskrit saying declares, "For yesterday is only a dream and tomorrow is but a vision . . . Look well, therefore, to this day." Choose to participate in today, be mindful, seek new interests—you can engage in your life as it is now, keeping your own story in mind. You still have the chance to write this chapter.

Living Well

- We are all a tiny part of this universe, and that can be both an overwhelming and a freeing thought. When faced with the reality that all of our lives are relatively brief, and we are indeed even physically tiny little specks in the universe, looking outside of yourself can allow you to move beyond isolation. If you are a believer of some sort, find comfort from your deity, or experience being connected with all the other bits of "stardust" who have peopled the earth. We are all tiny on our own, but as parts of the millennia of sentient life on earth we are massive.
- Loss is a part of life. Nobody looks forward to losing people, but running from the effects of loss is not possible or helpful. Allow memories to be a comfort and a way to keep a connection with those you've lost rather than focusing only on the pain.
- Grieving those we've lost honors them.
- The beauty of life is that we grow and change. Each episode, from cradle to grave, forms a rich tapestry. Allow yourself moments to appreciate what has been good, beautiful, and satisfying in your life.

PART THREE

moving beyond depression

10

seeking professional help

A self-help book or inspirational reading can be beneficial when you're experiencing depression. Sometimes, though, you need a helping hand. There is no shame in seeking help. Medications and medical treatments have provided relief from depression for many people. Many psychotherapies have documented positive outcomes for people living with depression. Getting the right support can be daunting. You may not know who you need to see: your medical doctor? A therapist? A religious leader? A friend? Navigating the path to care need not be a mystery, and here you can begin to chart the territory.

Considering Pharmaceutical Interventions

Many people living with depression can benefit from medication. Talking with a trained psychiatric practitioner about the best options for you can be valuable. The practice of psychopharmacology has evolved rapidly since the mid-20th century. New medications with fewer side effects, or formulations that can be combined to augment one another, continue to emerge.

Although you may have seen oversimplified commercials stating that your depression is caused by a chemical imbalance, it isn't as simple as that. The research is not clear that any one neurotransmitter (the "chemicals" in an "imbalance") causes depression. Plus, phrases like "depression is a serious medical illness" can either relieve you of feelings of guilt and shame or make you feel more stigmatized. The truth is that some medications treating psychological problems could benefit people without serious psychological problems—there is no "disease" required. So let's set aside the stigma around psychiatric medication.

But what if you're on medication that hasn't provided the relief you'd like? If so, you may need to discuss possible changes with a medical provider. Continuing with your current medication while adding some strategies from previous chapters may also help when medication alone isn't sufficient.

Antidepressants are not happy pills, and the benefits you receive from them may be subtle. They don't solve life problems, and they don't make the sun come out on gloomy days. They can, however, give you the wherewithal to look for solutions to your problems and provide a little more energy to enjoy the sunshine when it emerges. When they're not working as you'd like, there are therapies with strong research support in the treatment of depression.

Finding Psychotherapy Interventions

While not all therapies are equally supported by research, you can look to international guidelines to find evidence-based treatments. The strategies in this book have come from the cognitive and behavioral perspectives as described in the Introduction, but there may be other perspectives that resonate with you. Finding a skilled therapist who is well-trained in those perspectives and with whom you can form a connection can make a significant difference.

People often think about therapy as sitting with a therapist and telling them all your problems while that person provides some form of insight or asks repeatedly, "How did that make you feel?" This is a stereotype. Finding a counselor who fits this stereotype is not a good fit when you're living with depression. You need more than someone to ask how you feel and empathize with how hard your life is. When you tell a mental health professional that you are depressed, anyone worth their salt should know how you feel, and understand how you're likely to feel in given situations. A good therapist will help you to manage the feelings by making changes in your thinking or behavior; improving interpersonal relationships; or practicing mindful presence.

There are thousands of therapists and counselors in practice, yet quality care is difficult to find in many parts of the world. While I can't recommend one type of therapy without knowing you and what's available, I can say with confidence: Look for a therapist who is more than "a good listener." Seek out someone trained in therapies for depression.

In the 1990s, the Society of Clinical Psychology (Division 12) of the American Psychological Association developed criteria for rating the strength of research on various psychotherapies. The therapies that have informed this book are rated as having modest to strong evidence by several organizations.

Generally speaking, therapists who work from an orientation that is cognitive, cognitive-behavioral, behavioral, mindfulness-based, interpersonal, emotion-focused, problem-solving, or some integration of those—or who do brief psychodynamic therapy—are likely to have solid training in research-backed treatments. This also holds for practitioners of acceptance and commitment therapy (ACT) or rational emotive behavior therapy.

Therapists may also work from an integrative, "case-conceptualization" model; typically these therapists integrate evidence from research to provide individualized care. In practice, most therapists, regardless of their therapeutic orientation, will draw on the broader psychotherapy literature—and this is a good thing. Be wary of therapists who seem to have no theoretical grounding.

FACTORS TO CONSIDER

The type of therapy is not the only important aspect of receiving quality mental health care. Research on psychotherapy goes beyond examining the treatment strategies or theories of change that have empirical support. There are other factors that predict positive outcomes in psychotherapy. Therapists often refer to these as "common factors"—so named because they cut across theoretical orientations and matter regardless of the type of therapy.

It may not surprise you that a important factor in achieving a positive outcome is the relationship you have with your therapist. The therapist–client relationship is unique. It's not like a friendship, although you may regard your therapist fondly. You should believe that your therapist understands you, and that the two of you agree on the nature of your problems and share goals for treatment.

You may at times disagree with your therapist. Therapists, even the most well-trained, can say the wrong thing, be too pushy on a topic, miss something important you say, or make any number of mistakes over the course of treatment. Therapists are human, and gaining education and credentialing doesn't make anyone perfectly attuned to each person they will work with. When this happens, you may have a negative reaction to your therapist. Don't avoid it. If you notice yourself feeling hurt, angered, or dismissed during a session, discuss it with your therapist. A skilled clinician will welcome your feedback and work to repair any rupture in the relationship. This doesn't mean the therapist will agree with everything you say or feel, but they should take your concerns seriously and work collaboratively with you to address them.

Another key factor is your own engagement in the therapeutic process. Therapy is not a passive experience where you sit back and let someone fix you. You need to be an active participant—completing homework assignments, practicing new skills like the ones in this book between sessions, and being honest about what works and what doesn't. The more you put into therapy, the more you're likely to get out of it.

Finally, consistency matters. Attending sessions regularly and giving the process time to work matters. While some people experience rapid improvement, for others it takes weeks or months. Don't give up too quickly. At the same time, if after several months you're not seeing any progress, discuss it with your therapist and consider whether a different approach or clinician might suit you better.

Seeking Professional Help Even When You Don't Feel Like It

"I've been in therapy before, and it didn't help."

This is a common experience, and it doesn't mean therapy won't work for you. There are several possible reasons. Perhaps the therapist wasn't a good match for you. Perhaps the type of therapy wasn't well-suited to treating depression. Perhaps you weren't ready at the time to engage fully. Or perhaps life circumstances made it difficult to follow through with treatment.

BE HONEST

You have another opportunity. You might benefit from being more direct with a new therapist about your previous experience and what didn't work, so they can tailor their approach accordingly. You can also share with a therapist what you're learning in this book and what's been helpful and what hasn't, so together you can develop more solutions that work for you.

"When should I see a therapist or doctor?"

Some people see their general practitioner only when they run a high fever or are vomiting uncontrollably; others see a doctor when they're slightly queasy. We're different in our reactions to physical symptoms, and the same is true for psychological symptoms.

LET GO OF THE STIGMA YOU MAY FEEL

Getting help before a problem gets unmanageable, whether predominantly physical or psychological, is always a good idea. You might believe that seeking professional help signals that you're "crazy." You might even believe that you need to manage your depression on your own, lest it prove you're weak and confirm some of your unhelpful thinking. Ideas like this stem from the social stigma surrounding psychological problems. Fortunately, this stigma is lessening as more people speak openly about their experiences. Particularly following the COVID-19 pandemic, people around the world have recognized that mental health is as important as any aspect of physical health and are therefore more empathetic toward those experiencing psychological difficulties.

"I can't afford therapy."

Cost is a significant barrier for many people. However, options exist. Many therapists offer sliding scale fees based on income. Community mental health centers often provide services at reduced cost. Some therapists hold group sessions, which are less expensive than individual sessions. Teletherapy and online therapy platforms have expanded access and often cost less than traditional in-person therapy.

Until recently, participating in clinical trials for psychotherapy required living near a large research facility, but the internet has expanded access here too. Usually, treatment is provided free of charge, or participants receive minimal reimbursement when participating in clinical research. This could be an option you haven't previously considered.

"What if I need to be in therapy for the rest of my life?"

In some cases, psychotherapists can function like primary care doctors. When you have a good relationship with one, you may see them periodically throughout your life. It is probably not necessary to be continuously in therapy, but it also is not unusual for people to return to therapy periodically when they need support.

CBT is usually a shorter-term therapy, and if you are working with a CBT therapist, you may have times when you see them for focused work on a particular difficulty and then take a break from therapy. Returning to therapy repeatedly, or engaging in longer-term therapy, does not mean you have failed. We generally don't think of psychotherapy as "curing" people, but rather as helping people develop different ways to cope. Seeking help when you need it, throughout your life, is always an opportunity.

REMEMBER THAT MOODS FLUCTUATE

People who have experienced severe depression sometimes develop a fear of becoming depressed again. If you're vigilant about any dip in mood, recognize that there are normal fluctuations. You will still sometimes feel down when difficult things happen, and that does not mean you're on the brink of a depressive episode. You may have days when you're in a low mood. On those difficult days, make an extra effort to follow your plan, engage in activities aligned with your values, evaluate the accuracy of your thoughts, and lean into the mood rather than try to avoid it. You can be "in a mood" and still engage with the important activities and people in your life.

REMEMBER THAT THERE IS NEVER A LAST HOPE

You can always consult with different providers of medical or psychological care when the help you're receiving isn't enough. Psychiatrists can suggest alternatives or additional treatments. Research is ongoing in psychotherapy and in psychopharmacology. New insights and possibilities for help are always on the horizon.

Living Well

- It's wise to find support when you need it. You go to the dentist when you have a toothache, and you can seek out a mental health professional when you're struggling with depression.
- Not everyone has the same access to care, but there are ways to maximize what's within reach. Teletherapy has expanded exponentially since the COVID-19 pandemic, and increasingly, mental health providers are gaining expertise in delivering services online.

- There is no one perfect therapy for everyone. We know a great deal about what makes therapy effective. It is first important that you find a therapist with whom you can have a solid relationship.
- Medications and safe medical procedures are options worth considering. You don't need to be on medication forever, and having a thoughtful discussion with a medical provider about the best course of action to address your depression is an important step in living well.

11

savoring the good times, staying present through the bad

When you're living with depression and you then have better days, it's a great relief. You may want to coast and hope the next episode is a long way off. What you've learned to do—having a different relationship to your feelings, thoughts, and behaviors—is worth practicing even when you are well. You can extend times when you're feeling better and build protection against future episodes by staying proactive even when the depression is at bay.

Consider a singer taking lessons. Every singer has a comfortable vocal range. With training, anyone can reach higher or lower notes that require specific techniques. Beginners carefully follow all the rules for challenging notes but sing without thinking when in their comfortable range. The result? Those easier notes sound less polished than the difficult ones they've worked hard to master. Likewise, during good times, engaging in activities may come easily—like hitting comfortable notes within your range—but you're building habits to sustain you when you don't feel as good. Practice savoring good times and making the most of them.

Using the skills you've learned so far allows you to live well even when life is challenging. This chapter covers appreciating the good times, building resilience, and maintaining habits that keep you living well during challenging times.

No matter how hard you've worked to overcome or live well with depression, you'll face challenges. When you've been depressed, your reaction to challenges may be to shut down or feel pulled back into the depths. But you can hang on. You may have blue moods or bouts of depression, but you can still live well. Like a singer who doesn't always hit the high notes, your natural voice needn't slip back into sounding like a bad karaoke performance if you maintain the vocal practices that make it beautiful.

Savoring the Good Times Even When You Don't Feel Like It

Mood-dependent behavior isn't only driven by bad moods. You can deliberately make the most of good times, anchoring yourself to these moments to sustain you in harder times. Acting from the outside in shouldn't make you feel like an automaton—it's a strategy for living a values-driven life.

"I feel good! Will this last?"

In Chapter 10 we discussed the fear of experiencing severe depression again. Moods fluctuate normally, and feeling down for a day or week doesn't mean you're in another depressive episode. Staying engaged and using helpful thinking skills keep you steady during down times.

A related concern is feeling good but uncertain whether to trust it. We can't always predict how long good feelings will last. Life's peak moments usually aren't permanent—otherwise they'd be plateaus, not peaks.

Worrying about whether a good mood will last is understandable when you have periods of depression, but it's also a guaranteed buzzkill. Think of enjoying a delicious dessert after a nice meal while thinking, with each bite, "I have less and less left, and it will all be gone soon." Focusing on having the dessert running out takes away the enjoyment of eating it. You can always enjoy this delicious treat again, so enjoy each bite now rather than thinking about when it will be gone.

Good moods and good times, like good desserts, are episodic enjoyments. If you ate a delicious dessert endlessly, you'd lose your taste for it and probably feel sick. If you only feel good moods, you'll become bored. Have you ever met someone who is always upbeat, or seen such a character in a movie? They're annoying. In the holiday movie *Elf,* Will Ferrell's character "Buddy" sounds ridiculous when he exclaims, "Smiling's my favorite!"

STAY IN THE MOMENT

Attending mindfully to all aspects of an enjoyable activity enhances your enjoyment. For example, if you're sitting on a beach on a warm day feeling relaxed, you can savor the experience by focusing on everything happening in the moment. Start with the feel of the beach blanket or chair you're sitting on. How does it feel on your legs, or if you're lying down, on your back and head? If your eyes are open, watch clouds drifting by or seabirds flying. If your eyes are closed, listen to the waves and the sounds of others enjoying the day, and breathe in the fresh salt air. Or watch the water and follow the waves.

During relaxing activities—whether outside or in your own home—your mind might wander with all sorts of thoughts, good and bad. Those thoughts can easily pull you out of the moment. On the beach, for example, if you're watching waves but thinking about needing to put gas in your car or worrying about an ill relative, those thoughts steal your momentary respite. Those may be important concerns, and they'll still be important after your relaxing break. Instead, bring your mind back to the sounds around you. Look for things that pull your attention to the activity. On the beach, look for patterns in the sand. Have something nice to eat or drink, like ice cream or iced tea. Make the good time a special moment, whether you're on vacation or in your daily routine.

"I feel guilty about having fun."

You might struggle to enjoy yourself because you feel guilty about doing so. There may be many reasons for this, and we discuss a few below. You may relate to them, or you may have different experiences. You can apply what you've discovered about having a different relationship to your emotions, thoughts, and actions and learn to enjoy yourself without guilt.

SURVIVOR GUILT

When we've been more fortunate than people we care about, we can feel guilty about enjoying what they can't. This happens for people who survive an epidemic or natural disaster when others don't. It can happen at a personal level when a loved one has died. Some circumstances make it harder to allow yourself enjoyment, like when the loved one who died was younger than you or was your child. You might have survivor guilt over financial or professional success when others you know haven't succeeded. In Chapter 9 we suggested asking yourself, "Why not me?" when something bad happens. This question also applies when something good happens.

We tend to think in just-world terms—that what happens to us is based on what we deserve. Those beliefs are challenged when bad things happen to good people or when good things happen to bad people. You don't need to be a bad person to wonder why you get things you don't deserve any more than others you love, who may have done more noble things or were more innocent.

Your enjoyment doesn't take anything away from anyone else—unless you've stolen something from them to have a good time. Since that's highly unlikely, denying yourself a good time because someone else can't have one only hurts you. It can feel like you're "rubbing it in their face" even if the person you're thinking of is no longer living. That's how our minds play tricks on us.

Guilt serves a purpose if it keeps us from hurting others or repeating bad behavior. Guilt over experiences that don't harm anyone else serves no purpose. While we may fully acknowledge the psychological reality of survivor guilt, that doesn't make it useful. If you feel guilty about having opportunities that someone else doesn't, consider creating opportunities for others. Find ways to honor the values of your lost loved one, or to help others who remind you of that person. In addition to easing your guilt, these actions offer a constructive outlet for your sadness.

BELIEVING THAT HAVING FUN IS EQUAL TO NOT TAKING LIFE SERIOUSLY

You've lived through rough times. When you're feeling good and have an opportunity to have fun, you might feel guilty because it seems out of sync with harsh realities—you may almost feel foolish.

As a child, did you ever do some silly acrobatics that an adult corrected you for because it wasn't the right place or time? Did you feel embarrassed, ashamed, a little guilty for being a goofball? Is that how you feel now whenever you have fun? You don't need to be dancing on a table with a lampshade on your head to feel guilty—merely enjoying a nice meal that you splurged on can make you feel like you've gone overboard when you're living with depression.

Just as you need sleep or rest after vigorous activity to let your body recover, you need time to enjoy yourself. When you've had a break from everything you're serious about, you can tackle problems more competently. Having fun, getting away from responsibilities, taking a break from concerns, may give you new ideas for solving problems or improving some task you're required to do. When you need to make a decision and someone advises you to sleep on it, taking the time may give you clarity. The same is true for having breaks from the seriousness of life.

BELIEVING YOU DON'T DESERVE IT

In the 1951 film adaptation of Charles Dickens's *A Christmas Carol,* Ebenezer Scrooge feels joyous after being visited by the three ghosts and says, "I don't deserve to be so happy." You might feel like this without being visited by ghosts, simply because you think that you're a bad person or that you've done bad things. Once again, we could put "Why not me?" on repeat. Having fun does not mean you aren't atoning for wrongdoing, or that you can't make restitution. Even if you can't shake the belief that you're a bad person, having fun won't make you a worse person, unless it comes at the expense of others.

"What do I do when I'm not depressed?"

You might have difficulty savoring the good times because you've been depressed for so long or so often that you don't know what to do when you aren't depressed. It might feel like you aren't being yourself. When we're distressed, it can cloud our memory, making us stop recalling better times, and then we assume we've always felt this way. This leads us to another tip for what you can do when you aren't depressed.

WRITE A LETTER TO YOURSELF

Find some nice stationery or a greeting card and write down how you're feeling right now. Describe objectively what it feels like not to be depressed. How are your thoughts different? What does it feel like to enjoy activities? What are you motivated to do?

Reminisce about pleasant experiences from the past. Describe them too. You can even try to recall the best time you had in each year of your life and write about what happened. Of course you may not remember every year of your life, especially your earliest years, but see if you can jog your memory. Doing this can also allow those good memories to sit beside any bad memories you may have of the same times in your life.

List enjoyable activities that you've engaged in, especially those that you may have been reluctant to do but did anyway. If you can write about something that felt at first like a challenge but that you ultimately completed, your words will serve as a reminder that you've overcome struggles before.

Finish your letter with a message of hope for your depressed self. This letter is meant to be a caring reminder that good times are possible for you. Your words to yourself can be a light in darker times and may even help prevent future depression.

Staying Present through the Bad Times Even When You Don't Feel Like It

You can also continue to live well even when you're feeling depressed. All of the strategies presented in previous chapters can help you to do so. A few things to keep doing when you're depressed or distressed are staying connected to your values, considering the outcomes of your actions, finding ways to make the world a little better, recognizing that there is a "you" beyond your mood, and imagining other possibilities for your life than endless depression.

"Being a depressed person keeps me from having a good life."

Acceptance and commitment therapy (ACT) encourages us to live in the moment, because waiting until some change occurs keeps us disconnected from life. Thinking you'll be content when you find the perfect *something* keeps you from practicing contentment right now—which is what contentment is all about—accepting and living with what we have in the moment.

Granted, being depressed may make it harder to enjoy things, but it calls for evaluating your thoughts and consciously trying to break out of brooding. Some days you may give in and pull the covers over your head, but you can still do things to have a good life. That may sound ironic, but it only follows the philosophy that a good life isn't determined by being free of suffering. You can live a good life with a chronic illness or disability, and you can live a good life with a mood disorder.

Believing that depression keeps you from living well is a trap, as is thinking of your identity in terms of depression. Would you want a health care provider who referred to everyone by their diagnosis? What would you think if you heard them say, "Here comes the broken ankle," "Ah, today I see diverticulitis," or "That's my chronic health worrier"? You'd rightly choose someone else—someone who sees you as a person, not a diagnosis. Likewise, choose yourself over your depression. Treat yourself as you want others to treat you, and you'll see beyond your depression.

TAKE CARE WITH THE LABELS YOU'RE USING

Just as labels we place on others affect how we think and feel about them, so do labels we place on ourselves. Labels can be limiting. When we label others, we expect them to live up to those labels, distorting our experience of the real people around us. That's how prejudice and stigma flourish. When we label ourselves, it creates expectations that can be a hindrance.

When you label yourself as a "depressed person," you imply that you always act in a depressed manner. If you label yourself as a kind person, you expect yourself to always act in kind ways. Yet we know that no one is *always* their label. Someone who is generally kind in their treatment of others can still get angry and make a rude gesture or tell someone off. Although you may be depressed, you can still do activities that run counter to the mood you feel. This is how you act from the outside in and may actually change your mood.

"Nothing really matters when I'm still depressed."

Everything you do has consequences. That may sound dramatic because we often use "consequence" to mean punishment, but it simply means an outcome that follows a behavior. The smallest action has consequences, like turning left instead of right on your way to the market; maybe your drive is a few minutes longer, or you happen to see a family enjoying a bike ride together. They're no big deal, but they're still consequences. Even what seem like inactions have consequences. When you decide to stay in bed long after an alarm rings, it may seem like you're doing nothing, but the choice you made was an action with consequences: You might feel more rested when you arise, or you may have missed seeing a neighbor whose illness had concerned you walking past your house looking well and recovered.

LEAN ON THE ABCS OF BEHAVIOR

Consider the ABCs described in Chapter 2. Whenever you think nothing matters, look at the antecedent, the behavior, and the consequence. Test the belief that nothing matters by doing something intentionally and observing the outcome. Smile at someone you pass on the street. If they smile back, your behavior had an impact on them. If they don't smile back, try again with someone else. There's no guarantee we'll always get an outcome we'd like.

If you're shy and don't want to do something interpersonal, consider putting something you don't mind getting rid of on your doorstep with a sign that says "Free." It might be a coffee mug or a small appliance you no longer use. Is it still there after 24 hours? If not, your action had consequences—you discarded something no longer useful to you and may have given someone else something they needed. Every action has consequences. Every action matters.

If you're thinking about the meaning of life—if it seems there's no ultimate purpose, no consequence at the very end, why bother?—return to Chapter 9. Practice making the moments count. Assess the ABCs and examine the consequences of your actions. Look at what matters and has meaning today among the people around you—not in the cosmos.

IMAGINE THE OUTCOME

Of course, you can't wish something into existence or say a magic word to get a particular outcome. Nevertheless, when you think nothing matters, you may be assuming either that there will always be a bad outcome no matter what you do, or that there is no reason to hope for something good when you're depressed. Try imagining an outcome that you would look forward to. Think about something good happening and allow yourself to daydream about it for a moment. Doing so may not only give you a moment of hopefulness, it may also make it more likely that you'll take actions to help bring that outcome about.

"It is hard to bear being present with these feelings."

Savoring good times is not as difficult as staying present during the bad. Anyone feeling depressed or feeling nothing at all would feel a strong pull to distract themselves or escape. Many of the ways you might distract yourself, however, can keep you tuned out from the world, which isn't helpful when you're depressed and the best advice is to engage. Worse yet, forms of distraction like drugs and alcohol have negative consequences.

You can stay present with mindful activities like taking a walk and noticing everything you see, hear, or smell along the way. You can also add things like music, the aroma of easy-to-bake cookies, or hot tea. While these practices may offer some distraction from negative thoughts or a blue mood, they keep you engaged in the here and now.

DO YOUR PART

Another option when you are depressed is to find simple ways to look outside your current situation while staying present. Thoughts from a depressed mode may say that the things you do don't make a difference; however, you can act contrary to those thoughts. Consider small gestures that make things better for the planet or for other people. They're easy to do and don't cost money. Look at it from the perspective of the ABCs we talked about earlier: Notice a small problem (antecedent), remedy it (behavior), and watch the change in that moment (consequence).

Try each day to make the world a little better:

- Recycle a can
- Use a reusable cup rather than paper
- Let someone have a seat on the subway or bus
- Invite a shopper with one or two items to go ahead of you in a grocery line
- Get a cup of water for a dog tied on the sidewalk on a summer day
- Share your umbrella with someone you know

The list isn't exhaustive, but the gestures are sound and intended to be a springboard for your own ideas. You can have purpose and make each day meaningful by acting consistently with your values.

Living Well

- Take advantage of times when you're feeling better to practice savoring the moment. Depression can interfere with feeling pleasure, but engaging in rewarding activities matters nevertheless.
- Pay attention to all aspects of good times, past and present. Look at photos to remind yourself of enjoyable adventures.

- Document your good times and keep a record to review during harder times. This can help counter the belief that you've always been or will always be depressed. You'll have written proof that there have been better times and that there can be better times ahead.
- Finding ways to have a good life in small moments can free you from feeling as if you're only surviving your existence.

12

a road map through depression

We've covered a lot of territory in this book. In this chapter, we won't cover new terrain. Rather, we will review the most important take-aways this book offers, giving you a road map of sorts. If you stall or get trapped by depression, return to this chapter for a quick summary. Ideally, you can get back onto your path to living well with depression.

Be sure to also review the additional materials found online at *www.guilford.com/martell3-materials* for a list of books written by leading clinicians and researchers. Hearing similar recommendations in different voices may help you better relate to the messages. The way to provide a road map through depression is to go step by step and address the many ways you may feel stuck on the journey toward living well with depression.

Going Back to the Start: How Can You Live Well with Depression?

The first two strategies we presented were to accept your emotions and learn to have a different relationship with them. The idea of accepting depression may go against everything you've been taught and your own desire to feel better. It's legitimate to want to feel better. As we discuss in detail in Chapter 1, emotions and moods are tricky, and when we don't want to feel them, they pull us further in. For instance, you may relate to the experience of becoming depressed about being depressed. Or you may find that when your mood improves, you experience anxiety about becoming depressed in the future and feel low about it. This experience is common, particularly for those who have lived with severe depressive episodes and chronic depression.

The experience of depression can be overpowering. In his poignant description of his own depression, *The Noonday Demon,* author Andrew Solomon writes that taking a shower was overwhelming, and the fear kept him in his bed. He writes, "Twelve steps, which sounded to me then as onerous as a tour through the stations of the cross."[1] All of the recommendations in this book recognize how hard it is to do what seem to be the simplest things.

William Styron, recounting his personal experience of recovering from severe depression in *Darkness Visible,* writes, "There, whoever has been restored to health has almost always been restored to the capacity for serenity and joy, and this may be indemnity enough for having endured the despair beyond despair."[2]

Matthew Johnstone, author of *I Had a Black Dog* and *Living with a Black Dog,* in which the black dog is depression, wrote that even though depression, represented by the black dog metaphor, was still in his life, he'd learned how to take control of the beast rather than being controlled by it.[3] You may have found the capacity for "serenity and joy", or your experience may be more like having a black dog always at your side. With the strategies provided throughout this book, you can develop an understanding of your depression.

How to Allow Your Emotions

Allowing the emotions or moods that feel negative to you, or allowing the loss of any feeling at all, is understandably challenging and probably feels impossible. Keep in mind that allowing is not the same as acquiescing. When we talk about allowing emotions—or as it is sometimes called, accepting—we mean to let the emotion be and to continue to live life. It doesn't mean making friends with depression, nor does it mean pretending to be happy in the midst of feeling pain.

Andrew Solomon, writing from his personal experience, rightly states that "The opposite of depression is not happiness but vitality." He further states that his life "is vital, even when sad."[4] To continue living with vitality, you need to move forward rather than standing still.

In Chapter 1 we presented the concept of a values-driven life. This idea has been most clearly articulated by the developers of ACT. Think of your road map as steering you in the direction of your values—what's important to you in your relationships, work life, leisure, and, if you will, the spiritual or philosophical aspects of your life.

You can allow your feelings when you take action according to what you value rather than following the dictates of your mood. You'll recall that another way of saying this is acting from the outside in—you act according to what you value and the goals that fit those values, with the hope that over time those actions may change how you feel.

Some examples: You can feel anxious about speaking up at a public meeting and still speak, even if your voice is shaky. You can bite your tongue instead of lashing out at someone to keep from intensifying an argument. You may have felt intense grief and still attended the funeral of a dear loved one, even when your impulse was to stay away. You may even have had physical reactions like a stomachache before heading to the service, but you attended nevertheless.

The catch is that if you're trying to take action to feel better—to find a way to avoid the mood or feelings—those negative feelings are more likely to keep you in their grip.

Just as we're told to breathe through the discomfort when engaging in physical therapy, turning our attention to the breath can also help in emotionally challenging moments. While the breath isn't the answer to everything, it's a natural way to center yourself and stay in the moment, neither fleeing from the emotion nor responding to immediate impulses to act. You've probably heard people say they count to 10 when they get angry (before responding), and focusing on your breathing is another way to gather yourself and calm your central nervous system.

On the other hand, when you don't really feel anything, or at least nothing you can name, allowing that feeling can be harder. Feeling nothing is not uncommon in depression. In this case, the advice is modified slightly; instead we say: Act despite the mood.

This is not easy, and you need to act from the outside—in other words, by using external supports. The most logical supports are other people. If you can, identify one or two people to whom you can reach out in the hardest of times. What are you willing to discuss with them? Can you tell them when you're struggling? Can you also listen to them in their own struggles? If you can do this, you can also request their help, whether to come to your house and help you out of bed or accompany you when an outing feels particularly frightening.

How to Be Proactive

Of course, not everyone has someone they can rely on. You'll need to be proactive in getting the support you need. An external support can be a schedule (see Chapter 2), calendar, or a few things on a to-do list. They will help keep track of how activity affects your mood; you can note how you feel when you complete an activity. Does it give you a sense of accomplishment? Was it pleasurable? Did it move the dial one step further toward reaching a goal?

The scheduled activities may be relatively trivial and unlikely to make a big shift in your mood. In this situation, note how you feel at the beginning of the day before doing the activity, and then at the end of the day, once you've checked it off your list. Even if your feelings have shifted from "dread" to "relief," it's a positive shift. You're getting ahead of your feelings rather than letting your feelings (or lack of feelings) remain in the driver's seat.

You can also return to the letter you wrote in Chapter 11 when you feel at your worst. This can remind you that times can be good again, and that moods are temporary. When reading a letter you had written to yourself when you were feeling well, allow yourself to visualize the moment you were writing. As you bring this time to mind, you may also be brought back into that better place, if only briefly. You can acknowledge that your mood has lifted and that it will likely do so again.

How to Change Your Relationship to Your Thoughts

Having negative biases—what is commonly referred to as always seeing the glass as half empty—can make depression seem as if it's a never-ending cycle. You may have a tendency to ruminate over things, or to have "distortions" or unhelpful thoughts. As part of the road map through depression, being able to decenter from your thoughts in order to evaluate the accuracy of your beliefs and perceptions—or to defuse from your thoughts so that they don't pull you away from living your life in accordance with your values—is key to living well with depression.

Decentering is a central feature in cognitive therapy for depression. As we discussed in Chapter 3, decentering is simply being able to look objectively at your thoughts, to evaluate them as if from an outsider's view. This allows you to look for evidence of whether your perception or belief is likely to be as accurate as you think.

There is probably always some grain of truth, or at least some likelihood, in your thoughts. For example, if you think, "Those people are looking at me and judging me" when you see a group of young people huddled together on a street corner, it may be true that they've looked at you, and it's possible that some of them had a judgmental thought about you or even made a judgmental comment about you. But is it definitely true that all of them were looking at you with more than a glance in your direction, and that they were all concerned enough to have any thought about you at all?

Considered in this way, the likelihood that they were looking at you in judgment becomes rather low. And even if they did both of those things, so what? They aren't the boss of you! So, decentering allows you to evaluate your thoughts, to test your beliefs by running experiments to see if the hypotheses you form about yourself, others, and the future are confirmed, or if a less negative alternative might be true instead.

Defusing is similar, but with a twist. Defusing from your thoughts means getting them out from under your skin. A belief such as "I am unlovable" may feel real to you. It seems believable because there are years of conditioning to get it "under your skin." Defusion turns that "feels-like-it-is-part-of-me" thought into just what it is: words in your head that pull you away from living your life according to what you value.

Psychologist Steve Hayes uses the metaphor that these thoughts are like monsters on a bus making a lot of noise and pulling your attention away from driving the bus. When you defuse from them, you can stay in control of the bus while those monsters yell "Boo" as loudly and angrily as they like. It's only noise.

Finally, staying present can help you if you tend to brood and ruminate. Take your attention away from the rumination to see the colors and shapes, to feel the movement of your body through space, to hear the sounds around you, to smell the air and aromas around you. Or simply focus on your breathing, breathing in through your nose, sensing the coolness of the air as it enters your nostrils, feeling it fill your chest and belly, and then exhale through your mouth, releasing your worries, ruminations, and anxieties with each exhale.

The Simplified Road Map

In Part Two of the book, we presented ideas for dealing with various aspects of life, such as family and work or school. Consider those chapters tools to return to when you need encouragement for navigating difficulties. The three principles or strategies of allowing your emotions, being proactive, and thinking flexibly are the core tools that make the road map complete.

When you identify the kind of life you want to live, the life you value, you can ask yourself if you're living in a values-driven way. For example, if you value learning, you can explore many ways to discover new things, from reading books and watching how-to videos to listening to autobiographical podcasts and attending talks at your local library.

If you enjoy eating, you might simply check out what someone else has in their grocery cart and imagine what they're making, or watch a reel of someone cooking an interesting dessert. Consider actions consistent with your values. These are steps forward on the road map through depression—and possibly, little by little, out of it.

Living well with depression is not a linear process. You may have times when there is a strong pull to escape or avoid your feelings, yet allowing your feelings is exactly what's needed. At other times, you may be stuck in rumination, and if you have a thought that you can examine, great, but if examining the thought keeps you ruminating over it, you can try mindful breathing to stay in the moment and out of your head, or you can remind yourself that you're "having a thought" but that you are not that thought.

There is no fixed end goal, although what you value is your North Star. As you live according to your values, you will move among the processes of allowing emotion, staying present, acting proactively, and examining your thoughts.

My Hope for You

I'm aware that, throughout this book, words like "simple" and "small" have been used for encouragement. I acknowledge that these words do not mean that living well with depression is easy. It's not. Living well is not easy in general, but it's achievable. I have shared in the experience of many people living through this process, taking steps forward—and backward—despite overwhelming circumstances and desperate desires for it all to stop.

Life can also have many rewards. To use the word "simple" one more time, perhaps the best way to live well with depression is to relish all the simple things in life. Take time to taste the food you eat. Look for something that strikes you as pretty on your way to work or running errands. Remember a kindness someone did for you. The counterbalance to the truth that life is hard is that life is filled with marvels and beauty. It might take initial willingness to look for an alternative to a strongly held but unhelpful belief and to take the first steps in acting in a way consistent with your values even when you're feeling sad, anxious, or otherwise distressed. In the introduction, I said to start with hope. To close, let's end with an encouragement to hope and to practice living well. I share this hope with you.

notes

Introduction: A Day in the Life of Depression

1. Styron, W. (1992). *Darkness visible: A memoir of madness.* New York: Vintage.
2. American Psychiatric Association. (2022). *Diagnostic and statistical manual of mental disorders* (5th ed., text rev.). Washington, DC: American Psychiatric Association.
3. Styron, W. (1992). *Darkness visible: A memoir of madness* (p. 83). New York: Vintage.
4. Greenberger, D., & Padesky, C. A. (2016). *Mind over mood: Change how you feel by changing the way you think* (2nd ed.). New York: Guilford Press.
5. Jacobson, N. S., Martell, C. R., & Dimidjian, S. (2001). Behavioral activation therapy for depression: Returning to contextual roots. *Clinical Psychology: Science and Practice, 8*(3), 255–270.
6. Hayes, S. C., Strosahl, K. D., & Wilson, K. G. (2012). *Acceptance and commitment therapy: The process and practice of mindful change* (2nd ed.). New York: Guilford Press.
7. Weissman, M. M., Markowitz, J. C., & Klerman, G. L. (2017). *The guide to interpersonal psychotherapy* (updated and expanded ed.). Oxford, UK: Oxford University Press.

Chapter 1. Emotions: Allow Your Feelings

1. Barlow, D. H., Sauer-Zavala, S., Farchione, T. J., Urray Latin, H., Ellard, K. K., Bullis, J. R., et al. (2018). *Unified protocol for transdiagnostic treatment of emotional disorders* (2nd edition). Oxford, UK: Oxford University Press.
2. Iglesias-González, M., Aznar-Lou, I., Peñarrubia-Maria, M. T., Gil-Girbau, M., Fernández-Vergel, R., Alonso, J., et al. (2018). Effectiveness of watchful waiting versus antidepressants for patients diagnosed of mild to moderate depression in primary care: A 12-month pragmatic clinical trial (INFAP study). *European Psychiatry, 53,* 66–73.
3. Brown, G. S. (2023, May 19). Happiness is fleeting. Aim for fulfillment. *Washington Post. www.washingtonpost.com/wellness/2023/05/19/fulfilled-life-happiness-strategies.*

Chapter 2. Behaviors: Be Proactive

1. Rhodes, S., Richards, D. A., Ekers, D., McMillan, D., Byford, S., Farrand, P., et al. (2014). Cost and outcome of behavioural activation versus cognitive behavioural therapy for depression (COBRA): Study protocol for a randomized controlled trial. *Trials, 15,* 29.
2. Aupperle, R., Smith, R., Kirlic, N., McDermott, T., Akeman, E., Santiago, J., et al. (2019). A computational, approach-avoidance framework for predicting behavioral therapy response for generalized anxiety disorder and major depressive disorder. *Neuropsychopharmacology, 44*(Supplement 1), 397–398.

Chapter 3. Thoughts: Think Flexibly

1. Beck, A. T. (1967). *Depression: Causes and treatment.* Philadelphia: University of Pennsylvania Press.
2. Young, J. E., & Klosko, J. (1993). *Reinventing your life.* New York: Dutton.
3. Hayes, S. C. (2025). *Get out of your mind and into your life: The new acceptance and commitment therapy* (20th anniversary edition). Thousand Oaks, CA: New Harbinger.

Chapter 4. Keeping Up with Self-Care

1. Ellis, A. E., & Harper, R. A. (1975). *A guide to rational living.* Chatsworth, CA: Wilshire.

Chapter 7. Thriving with a Partner

1. Christensen, A., & Heavey, C. L. (1990). Gender and social structure in demand/withdraw pattern of marital conflict. *Journal of Personality and Social Psychology, 59*(1), 73–81.
2. Gottman, J., Notarius, C., Gonso, J., & Markman, H. (1979). *A couple's guide to communication.* Champaign, IL: Research Press.

Chapter 8. Engaging with School, Work, and Hobbies

1. Doran, G. T. (1981). There's a SMART way to write management's goals and objectives. *Journal of Management Review, 70,* 35–36.

Chapter 9. Considering What's Greater Than You

1. Yousefi, N. (2024, December 4). Journeys to humanism: Finding meaning in aiding others. *The Humanist. https://thehumanist.com/magazine/fall-2024/up-front/journeys-to-humanism-finding-meaning-in-aiding-others.*
2. Kushner, H. S. (1981). *When bad things happen to good people* (page 10). New York: Macmillan.
3. Vonnegut, K., Jr. (1968). *Slaughterhouse-five* (pages 76–77). New York: Dell.
4. Statista. (2026). *Global wealth distribution in 2024, by net worth of individuals.* Retrieved March 10, 2026, from *www.statista.com/statistics/203930/global-wealth-distribution-by-net-worth.*
5. Sybertz, A. (2026). This is one of the rarest facial features in the world. *Reader's Digest.* Retrieved from March 11, 2026, from *www.rd.com/article/different-colored-eyes.*

6. Statista. (2026). *Global wealth distribution in 2024, by net worth of individuals.* Retrieved March 10, 2026, from *www.statista.com/statistics/203930/global-wealth-distribution-by-net-worth.*

Chapter 12. A Road Map through Depression

1. Solomon, A. (2001). *The noonday demon: An atlas of depression* (page 53). New York: Scribner.
2. Styron, W. (1992). *Darkness visible: A memoir of madness* (page 84). New York: Vintage.
3. Johnstone, M. (2005). *I had a black dog.* Sydney: Pan MacMillan Australia.
4. Solomon, A. (2001). *The noonday demon: An atlas of depression* (page 443). New York: Scribner.

index

about the author

Christopher R. Martell, PhD, ABPP, is Professor of Practice in the Department of Psychological and Brain Sciences at the University of Massachusetts Amherst. He is also Clinic Director at the Psychological Services Center, the training clinic for doctoral students at UMass. Previously, Dr. Martell had a private practice in Seattle for over 20 years. He has trained and supervised clinicians and provided research consultation around the world, with a focus on behavioral activation treatment for depression.